About the NCCN Guidelines for Patients®

NCCN National Comprehensive Cancer Network®

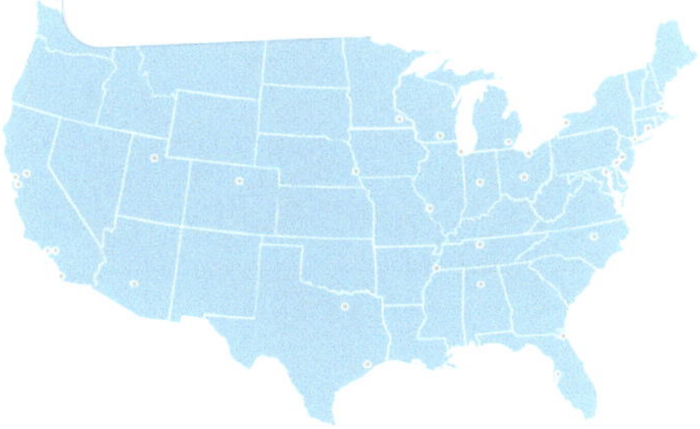

Did you know that top cancer centers across the United States work together to improve cancer care? This alliance of leading cancer centers is called the National Comprehensive Cancer Network® (NCCN®).

Cancer care is always changing. NCCN develops evidence-based cancer care recommendations used by health care providers worldwide. These frequently updated recommendations are the NCCN Clinical Practice Guidelines in Oncology (NCCN Guidelines®). The NCCN Guidelines for Patients plainly explain these expert recommendations for people with cancer and caregivers.

These NCCN Guidelines for Patients are based on the NCCN Clinical Practice Guidelines in Oncology (NCCN Guidelines®) for Head and Neck Cancers Version 1.2024 – October 9, 2023.

View the NCCN Guidelines for Patients free online
NCCN.org/patientguidelines

Find an NCCN Cancer Center near you
NCCN.org/cancercenters

Connect with us

Supporters

NCCN Guidelines for Patients are supported by funding from the NCCN Foundation®

To make a gift or learn more, visit online or email

NCCNFoundation.org/donate

PatientGuidelines@NCCN.org

Contents

NCCN Foundation seeks to support the millions of patients and their families affected by a cancer diagnosis by funding and distributing NCCN Guidelines for Patients. NCCN Foundation is also committed to advancing cancer treatment by funding the nation's promising doctors at the center of innovation in cancer research. For more details and the full library of patient and caregiver resources, visit NCCN.org/patients.

National Comprehensive Cancer Network (NCCN) and NCCN Foundation
3025 Chemical Road, Suite 100, Plymouth Meeting, PA 19462 USA

1

Throat cancer basics

The throat is located in the back of the mouth and in the neck. Cancer can form in part of the throat called the oropharynx. The oropharynx includes the back of the roof of the mouth (soft palate), the tonsils, the side and back walls of throat, and the base of the tongue.

The throat

The throat is a hollow, muscular tube inside the neck that starts behind the nose and ends at the top of the trachea (windpipe) and esophagus (the tube that goes to the stomach). The throat acts as a passageway for air to enter the lungs and food and liquid to enter the esophagus. It contains many structures, including the tonsils, pharynx, and larynx.

Some important structures of the throat and mouth:

- **Oral cavity** is another name for mouth.
- **Hard palate** is the hard, front part of the roof of the mouth behind the teeth.
- **Soft palate** is the soft, back part of the roof of the mouth.
- **Tongue** includes several muscles that extend from your hyoid bone (located in the middle of your neck) to the floor of your mouth.
- **Pharynx** is the throat.
- **Larynx** is a specific part of the throat also known as the voice box.
- **Esophagus** is a hollow muscular tube that carries food and liquid to the stomach.
- **Trachea** or windpipe leads to the lungs.

The pharynx

The pharynx is part of the throat and starts behind the nose (nasal cavity) and opens into the larynx and esophagus.

The pharynx (said fair-inks) has 3 parts:

- Nasopharynx
- Oropharynx
- Hypopharynx

Cancer can be found in any part of the pharynx. This book will focus on cancer of the oropharynx and will refer to the oropharynx as the throat. The oropharynx includes the back of the roof of the mouth (soft palate), the tonsils, the side and back walls of the throat, and the base of the tongue found in the throat.

The oropharynx

The oropharynx includes the back of the roof of the mouth (soft palate), the tonsils, the side and back walls of the throat, and the back (base) of the tongue. This book will refer to the oropharynx as the throat.

Parts of the Oropharynx

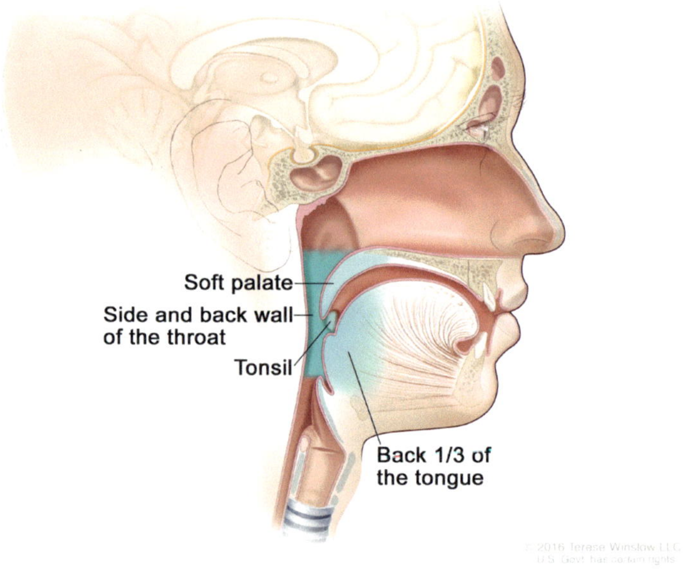

The pharynx

The pharynx is a hollow, muscular tube inside the neck that starts behind the nose and opens into the larynx and esophagus. The pharynx has 3 parts: the nasopharynx, oropharynx, and hypopharynx.

Anatomy of the Pharynx

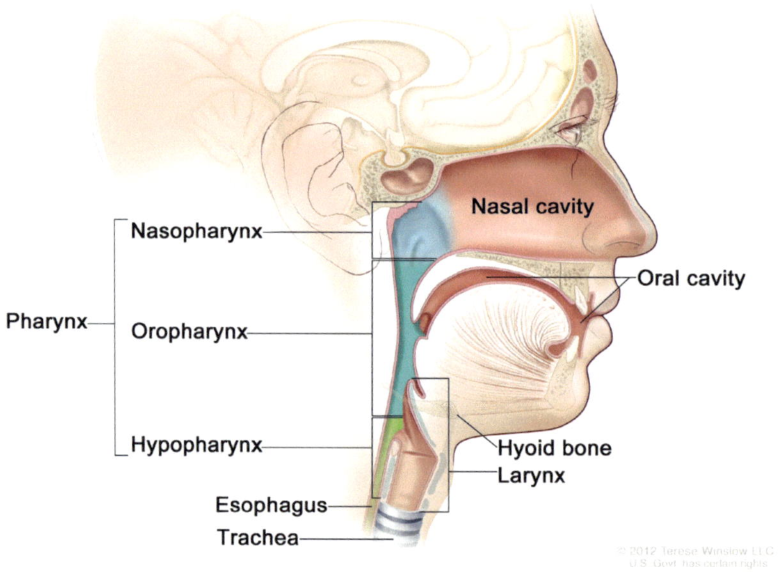

Head and neck cancers

Head and neck cancers are a group of cancers that arise in the head or neck area of the body. Cancer is named and treated based on the tumor location or where the cancer started.

Cancer can occur in the:

- Mouth (oral cavity),
- Middle part of the throat near the mouth (oropharynx),
- Space behind the nose (nasal cavity and paranasal sinuses),
- Upper part of the throat near the nasal cavity (nasopharynx),
- Voice box (larynx), or
- Lower part of the throat behind the larynx (hypopharynx).

Squamous cell carcinoma of the head and neck (SCCHN or HNSCC) is the most common type of head and neck cancer. It forms in the thin, flat cells of the mucus membranes of the mouth (oral), nose (nasal), and throat (pharynx). Mucus is a thick, slippery fluid. Squamous cells are found throughout the body, including the skin.

It is strongly recommended, when possible, for those with head and neck cancer to be treated at a high-volume center or hospital that has experience in their type of cancer.

More information on mouth cancer and nasopharyngeal cancer can be found at NCCN.org/patientguidelines and on the NCCN Patient Guides for Cancer app.

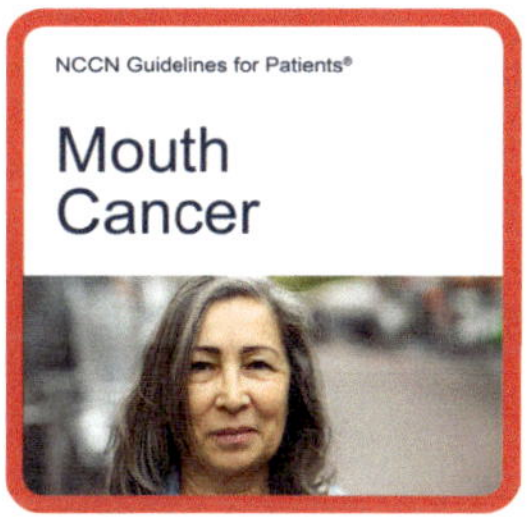

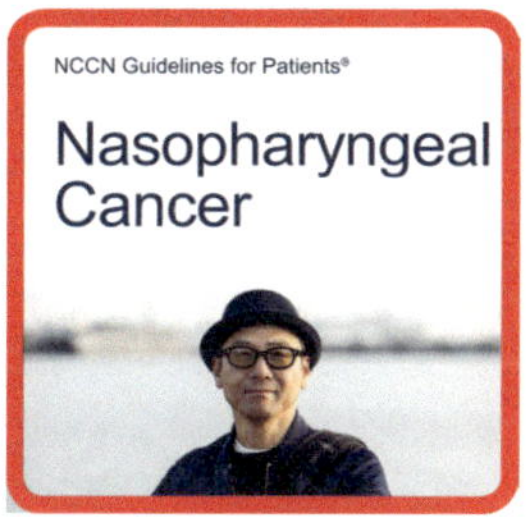

Throat cancer

Throat cancer starts in the oropharynx. Squamous cell carcinoma (SCC) is the most common type of throat cancer and is the focus of this book.

Cancer cells form a tumor called a primary tumor within the area of the oropharynx. This area includes the back of the roof of the mouth (soft palate), the tonsils, the side and back walls of throat, and base of the tongue. Tumors can grow into nearby tissue and organs, such as the voice box (larynx). Cancer cells often spread to lymph nodes in the neck, and less frequently, the lungs, liver, or spine.

Key points

- Head and neck cancers are a group of cancers that arise in the head or neck area of the body.
- Squamous cell carcinoma of the head and neck (SCCHN or HNSCC) forms in the thin, flat cells of the mucus membranes of the mouth (oral), nose (nasal), and throat (pharynx).
- Most head and neck cancers are squamous cell carcinomas (SCCs). SCC of the throat (oropharynx) is the focus of this book.
- The oropharynx includes the back of the roof of the mouth (soft palate), the tonsils, the side and back walls of throat, and base of the tongue found in the throat.

2
Testing for throat cancer

Treatment planning starts with testing. This chapter presents an overview of the tests you might receive and what to expect.

Test results

Results from imaging studies and a biopsy will be used to determine your treatment plan. Treatment will be based on these findings. It is important you understand what these tests mean. Ask questions and keep copies of your test results. Online patient portals are a great way to access your test results. Please discuss your results with your health care provider.

Keep these things in mind:

- Choose a friend, family member, or peer who can drive you to appointments, provide meals, or offer emotional support during diagnosis and treatment.
- Bring someone with you to doctor visits, if possible.
- Write down questions and take notes during appointments. Don't be afraid to ask your care team questions. Get to know your care team and help them get to know you.
- Get copies of blood tests, imaging results, and reports about the specific type of cancer you have.
- Organize your papers. Create files for insurance forms, medical records, and test results. You can do the same on your computer.
- Keep a list of contact information for everyone on your care team. Add it to your phone. Hang the list on your refrigerator or keep it in a place where someone can access it in an emergency. Keep your primary care physician (PCP) informed of changes to this list. You are encouraged to keep your PCP in the loop. They are great partners in your care.
- In your contact list, include information on the exact type of cancer, as well as any treatments and the date each treatment started.

For possible tests, **see Guide 1**.

General health tests

Some general health tests are described next.

Medical history

A medical history is a record of all health issues and treatments you have had in your life. Be prepared to list any illness or injury and when it happened. Bring a list of old and new medicines and any over-the-counter (OTC) medicines, herbals, or supplements you take. Some supplements interact with and affect medicines that your care team may prescribe. Tell your care team about any symptoms you have. A medical history, sometimes called a health history, will help determine which treatment is best for you.

Family history

Head and neck cancers are not inherited from your biological parents. However, some cancers and other diseases can run in families. Your care team will ask about the health history of family members who are blood relatives. This information is called a family history. Ask family members on both sides of your family about their health issues like heart disease, cancer, and diabetes, and at what age they were diagnosed. It's important to know the specific type of cancer or where the cancer started, if it is in multiple locations, and if they had genetic testing.

Guide 1 Tests for treatment planning
Biopsy of main tumor with human papillomavirus (HPV) testing by p16
Medical history, tobacco and alcohol use history, and physical exam, including complete head and neck exam. Mirror and fiberoptic exam if needed. Screen for depression.
CT scan with contrast and/or MRI with or without contast of main tumor and neck
As needed: • Endoscopy with examination under anesthesia (EUA) • Pre-anesthesia exam • FDG-PET/CT • Chest CT (with or without contrast) • Dental exam and x-ray (Panorex) • Nutrition, speech, and swallowing evaluation, and hearing test (audiogram) • Help to quit smoking • Fertility counseling • Screening for hepatitis B

Tobacco and alcohol use history

Tobacco and alcohol use are known risk factors for developing head and neck cancer and can limit how well treatment works.Their use can affect survival. You will be asked about your tobacco and alcohol use history and asked to avoid tobacco and limit alcohol use during treatment. Speak to your care team if you have any questions or concerns.

Physical exam

During a physical exam, your health care provider may:

- Check your temperature, blood pressure, pulse, and breathing rate
- Check your height and weight
- Listen to your lungs and heart
- Look in your eyes, ears, nose, and throat
- Feel and apply pressure to parts of your body to see if organs are of normal size, are soft or hard, or cause pain when touched.
- Feel for enlarged lymph nodes in your neck, underarm, and groin.

Complete head and neck exam

A physical exam will include the head and neck. Since the oropharynx is found inside the throat, some parts are not easy to see when your mouth is open. A doctor might use a special mirror or fiberoptic scope passed through your mouth or nose to look at these areas.

Dental exam

It is important to tell your dentist about your head and neck cancer and to have regular dental cleanings and checkups. Head and neck cancer and its treatment can affect the health of your jaw, teeth, and gums. If you need any dental work or procedures, they might be recommended before starting certain treatment.

Distress screening

It is normal to have strong feelings about being diagnosed with cancer, and your feelings can change from day to day and week to week. Talk to your care team and those whom you feel most comfortable about how you are feeling. There are services and people who can help you. Support and counseling are available. Many treatment teams include mind and body therapists who can help.

Dealing with a cancer diagnosis can be stressful and may cause further distress. Distress is an unpleasant experience of a mental, physical, social, or spiritual nature. It can affect how you feel, think, and act. Distress might include feelings of sadness, fear, helplessness, worry, anger, and guilt. You may also experience depression, anxiety, and sleep issues. Your treatment team will screen your level of distress. This is part of your cancer care.

Hearing test

A hearing test shows if there is any hearing loss, and if so, the type of hearing loss, how severe it is, and what might have caused it. An audiogram is a graph showing the results of a pure-tone hearing test. Tumors in the head and neck can affect hearing. Treatment of head and neck tumors can also affect hearing.

Hepatitis B and hepatitis C screening

Hepatitis B (HBV) and hepatitis C (HCV) are types of liver disease caused by a virus. A hepatitis blood test will tell your treatment team if you had hepatitis in the past or if you have it today. Some cancer treatments can wake up (or reactivate) the virus. If this happens, it can cause harm to the liver.

Lung function tests

Lung function tests or pulmonary function tests (PFTs) measure how well the lungs work. They measure how much air the lungs can hold and how quickly air is moved into and out of the lungs. They also measure how much oxygen is used and how much carbon dioxide is given off during breathing.

Nutrition assessment

You should meet with a nutrition expert before starting treatment. A nutritionist or dietician can suggest the best foods and fluids for you. It is important that you receive adequate and sustained nutrition before you start treatment. During and after treatment, your treatment team will monitor you for weight loss and other signs you aren't receiving enough nutrition.

If you smoke or vape, seek help to quit

A history of smoking or vaping nicotine increases your chances of developing head and neck, lung, and other cancers. Smoking and vaping can limit how well cancer treatment works and prevent wound healing. They also greatly increase your chances of having side effects during and after surgery. Cannabis use might also affect the amount of anesthesia used during surgery.

Nicotine is the chemical in tobacco that makes you want to keep smoking and vaping. Nicotine withdrawal is challenging for most people who smoke or vape. The stress of having cancer may make it even harder to quit. If you smoke or vape, ask your care team about counseling and medicines to help you quit. In head and neck cancers, stopping smoking or vaping is essential to maximize the chance for cure and minimize side effects.

For online support, try these websites:

- SmokeFree.gov
- BeTobaccoFree.gov
- CDC.gov/tobacco

Performance status

Performance status (PS) is a person's general level of fitness and ability to perform daily self-care tasks. Your state of general health will be rated using a PS scale called Eastern Cooperative Oncology Group (ECOG). PS is one factor taken into consideration when choosing a treatment plan. Your preferences about treatment are always important. The ECOG PS scores range from 0 to 5.

- **PS 0** means the person is fully active.
- **PS 1** means the person is still able to perform light to moderate activity, but with some limitations.
- **PS 2** means the person is limited to the chair or bed less than half of the time and is still able to care for self.
- **PS 3** means the person is limited to the chair or bed more than half of the time.
- **PS 4** means the person is totally confined to the bed or chair and completely unable to care for self.
- **PS 5** means the person is not alive.

In head and neck cancer, PS might be referred to as good or poor. Good PS is usually PS 0 or PS 1.

Pre-anesthesia exam

Anesthesia is loss of feeling or awareness caused by drugs. It keeps you from feeling pain from surgery or other procedures. A pre-anesthesia assessment will be done by the anesthesiologist. It will include a physical exam of your throat and airway. You be asked questions about your medical history, past surgery experiences, if you have any allergies to drugs or medicines, your understanding of the procedure, and how your appearance and function might change. Head and neck cancer surgery is complex. It is further complicated by other health conditions, airway and swallowing issues, tobacco and alcohol use, and tumor location. Being prepared and knowing what to expect after surgery will help prevent severe complications.

Fertility (all genders)

Treatment such as chemotherapy can affect your fertility, the ability to have children. If you think you want children in the future, ask your care team how cancer and cancer treatment might change your fertility. To preserve your fertility, you may need to take action before starting cancer treatment. Those who want to have children in the future should be referred to a fertility specialist to discuss the options before starting treatment.

Fertility preservation is all about keeping your options open, whether you know you want to have children later in life or aren't really sure at the moment. Fertility and reproductive specialists can help you sort through what may be best for your situation.

More information on fertility preservation is available at NCCN.org/patientguidelines and on the NCCN Patient Guides for Cancer app.

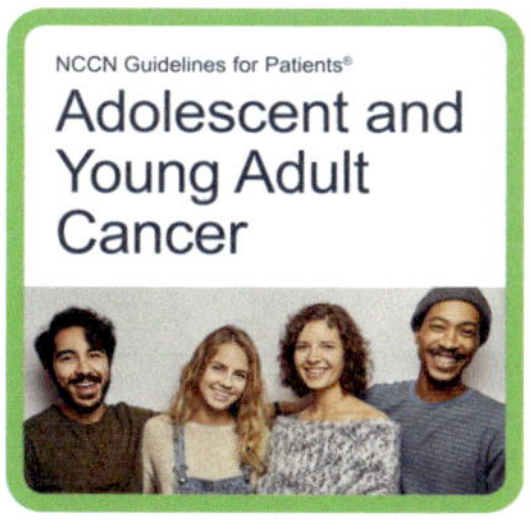

Changes in fertility

Treatment might cause your fertility to be temporarily or permanently impaired or interrupted. This loss of fertility is related to your age at time of diagnosis, treatment type(s), treatment dose, and treatment length. Talk to your care team about your concerns and if you are planning a pregnancy.

Preventing pregnancy during treatment

Preventing pregnancy during treatment is important. Cancer and cancer treatment can affect the ovaries and damage sperm. Hormonal birth control may or may not be recommended, so ask your doctor about options such as intrauterine devices (IUDs) and barrier methods. Types of barrier methods include condoms, diaphragms, cervical caps, and the contraceptive sponge.

Those with ovaries

Those who can become pregnant will have a pregnancy test before starting treatment. Cancer treatment can hurt the developing baby if you are or become pregnant during treatment. Therefore, birth control to prevent pregnancy during and after treatment is recommended. If you are pregnant or breastfeeding at the time of your cancer diagnosis, certain treatments will need to be avoided.

Menstruation, menses, menstrual flow, or your "period" may stop during treatment, but often returns within 2 years after treatment in those 35 years of age and under. It is still possible to become pregnant even though you might not have a period. Therefore, birth control is recommended during and after treatment. Consult your doctor for the best time to plan a pregnancy.

Those with testicles

Cancer and cancer treatment can damage sperm. Therefore, use contraception (birth control) such as condoms to prevent pregnancy during and immediately after cancer treatment.

p16 (HPV) testing

For throat cancer, biopsy samples are tested for the p16 protein to see if human papillomavirus (HPV) infection is present. This is a key part of staging (finding out if and how much the cancer has spread) and expected treatment results, and is considered when making treatment decisions. Cancers that are linked to HPV tend to respond better to treatment. p16 testing is different than HPV testing. p16 is used as a surrogate marker for HPV infection because p16 usually increases in cancer cells when HPV is present.

HPV

Human papillomavirus (HPV) is a group of viruses that infect the cells on the surface of skin or on the moist surfaces or inner linings of some organs and body cavities, such as the cervix, vagina, vulva, penis, anus, mouth, and throat. HPV infection usually clears on its own. However, HPV infections can cause abnormal tissue growth (warts) and sometimes cancer. Cancer caused by HPV is called HPV-related cancer.

HPV is the main cause of squamous cell carcinomas of the throat (oropharynx), particularly cancers of the tonsils and base of the tongue. HPV type 16 is responsible for 9 out of 10 throat cancers. The remaining cancers are caused by HPV18, 33, and 35. HPV-positive (HPV+) throat cancer is a distinct disease with specific tumor features that can be targeted during treatment.

p16

HPV16 is detected using a test to look for p16. p16 is a protein that slows cell division. It is produced by a gene located on chromosome 9 (shown as 9p21.3). Human cells have 23 pairs of chromosomes or 46 chromosomes in total. Testing to look for the presence (expression) of p16 is called biomarker testing. p16 can be found in cancers such as throat, cervical, vulvar, melanoma, and esophageal. When too much (overexpression) of p16 is found in throat cancer, it means that the cancer is usually caused by HPV. It might be written as p16+, HPV+, p16+/HPV+, or p16 (HPV)-positive. However, HPV+ cancer can be p16-. This might be written as p16-/HPV+.

Your preferences about treatment are always important. Talk to your care team and make your wishes known.

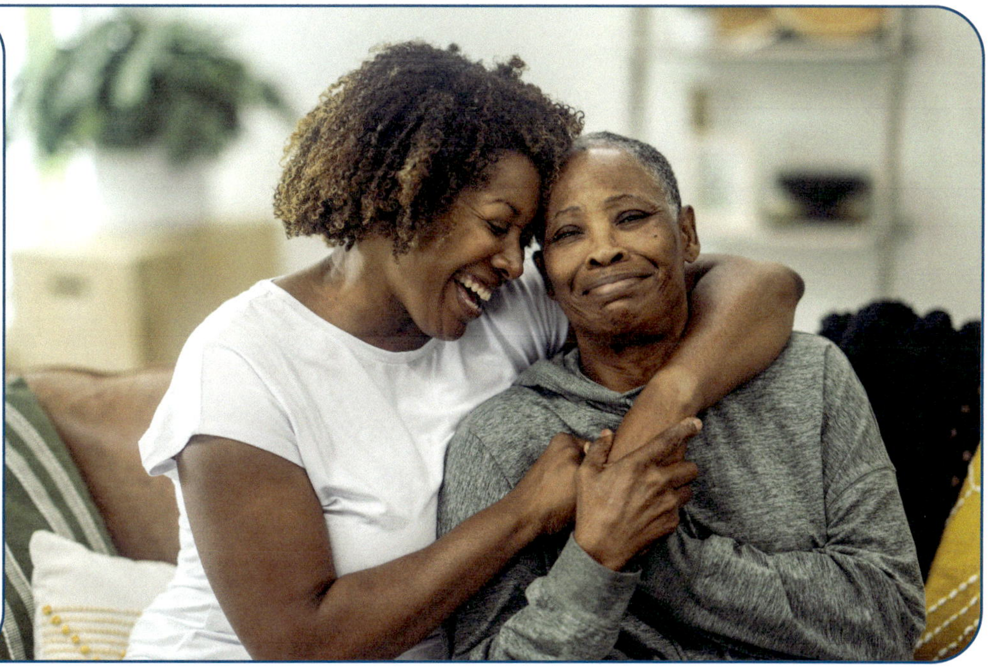

Imaging tests

Imaging tests take pictures of the inside of your body. Imaging tests show the primary tumor, or where the cancer started, and look for cancer in other parts of the body. A radiologist, an expert in interpreting imaging tests, will write a report and send this report to your health care provider (HCP). It is likely that the report will be sent directly to you through your patient portal or patient access system. You should discuss these results with your HCP. Some imaging tests are described next.

CT scan

A computed tomography (CT or CAT) scan uses x-rays and computer technology to take pictures of the inside of the body. A CT scan takes many x-rays of the same body part from different angles. All the images are combined to make one detailed picture. A CT scan of your neck and chest may be one of the tests to look for cancer. In most cases, contrast will be used.

MRI scan

A magnetic resonance imaging (MRI) scan uses radio waves and powerful magnets to take pictures of the inside of the body. It does not use x-rays and there is no radiation exposure. Because of the very strong magnets used in the MRI machine, tell the technologist if you have any metal in your body. During the test, you will likely be asked to hold your breath for 10 to 20 seconds as the technician collects the images. Contrast is often used.

A closed MRI has a capsule-like design where the magnet surrounds you. An open MRI has a magnetic top and bottom, which allows for an opening on each end. Closed MRIs are more common than open MRIs, so if you have claustrophobia (a dread or fear of enclosed spaces), be sure to talk to your care team about it.

Contrast material

Contrast material is used to improve the pictures of the inside of the body. Contrast materials are not dyes, but substances that help enhance and improve the images of several organs and structures in the body. It is used to make the pictures clearer. The contrast is not permanent and will leave the body in your urine immediately after the test. The types of contrast vary and are different for CT and MRI.

Tell your care team if you have had allergic reactions to contrast in the past. This is important. You might be given medicines to avoid the effects of those allergies. Contrast might not be used if you have a serious allergy or if your kidneys aren't working well.

PET scan

A positron emission tomography (PET) scan uses a radioactive sugar-based substance called a tracer. A tracer is injected into a vein to see where cancer cells are in the body and if they are using sugar produced by your body to grow. Cancer cells show up as bright spots on PET scans. However, not all tumors will appear on a PET scan. Also, not all bright spots are cancer. It is normal for the brain, heart, kidneys, and bladder to be bright on PET. Inflammation or infection can also show up as a bright spot. When a PET scan is combined with CT, it is called a PET/CT scan.

FDG-PET/CT

An FDG-PET/CT uses a radiotracer called F-18 fluorodeoxyglucose (FDG). It is made of fluoride and a simple form of sugar called glucose. You cannot eat or drink for at least 4 hours before the scan. This scan is most helpful when other imaging results are unclear. It may help identify cancer in primary sites, lymph nodes, and/or distant sites. If it clearly shows cancer in the bone, a bone scan and sodium fluoride PET/CT may not be needed. FDG-PET/CT can be done at the same time as a CT used for diagnosis.

Ultrasound

Ultrasound (US) uses high-energy sound waves to form pictures of the inside of the body. This is similar to the sonogram used for pregnancy. A wand-like probe (transducer) will be held and moved on your neck using gel. Ultrasound is painless and does not use x-rays, so it can be repeated as needed. Ultrasound is good at showing small areas of cancer that may be in lymph nodes. Sometimes, an ultrasound or CT is used to guide a fine-needle biopsy (FNB).

Keep these things in mind

- Take care of yourself. This is a stressful time. Seek out and ask for support. Support can be a friend, relative, neighbor, or coworker.
- This will be a confusing time. You will hear a lot of unfamiliar words. Interact with your health care team, ask questions, and talk about how you feel.

Panoramic dental x-ray

A panoramic dental x-ray or panoramic x-ray (Panorex) uses a very small dose of radiation to capture the entire mouth in one image, including the teeth, upper and lower jaw, and surrounding structures and tissues. It is commonly performed by dentists and oral surgeons in everyday practice and may be used to plan treatment for dentures, braces, extractions, and implants.

Scoping procedures

Some imaging tests use a thin, tube-shaped tool called a scope that is inserted into the mouth or nose body to examine the oropharynx and to take pictures. One end of the scope has a small light and camera lens to see inside your body. The image is sent to a television or computer monitor. This will also help guide your doctor in performing a biopsy.

More than one type of scope may be used for imaging tests. The type of scope often used for head and cancer is called an endoscope. An endoscope is often guided into the body through the mouth or nose. Endoscopy might be used to determine the size and spread of tumor and to take a tumor sample. Before an endoscopy, you will be given a topical spray to numb the throat.

Some possible endoscopies are described next. You might not have an endoscopy.

Fiberoptic nasopharyngolaryngoscopy

Fiberoptic nasopharyngolaryngoscopy is used to examine the larynx (voice box) and nearby structures. It is done while you are awake with a topical spray to make you more comfortable.

Laryngoscopy and nasolaryngoscopy

Laryngoscopy is an exam of the back of your throat, including your voice box (larynx) or behind your voice box (hypopharynx). It uses a laryngoscope, which is a thin, long tube fitted with a fiberoptic light. Your voice box contains your vocal cords and allows you to speak. A laryngoscope is used to look for tumors in the throat and voice box (larynx) and hypopharynx.

Laryngoscopy may be done in different ways:

- **Indirect laryngoscopy** uses a small mirror held at the back of your throat. The doctor shines a light on the mirror to view the throat area. Medicine to numb the back of your throat may be used.
- **Fiberoptic laryngoscopy (nasolaryngoscopy)** uses a small flexible scope passed through your nose and into your throat. Numbing medicine will be sprayed in your nose. This procedure typically takes less than 1 minute.
- **Direct laryngoscopy** is a more detailed exam performed under general anesthesia in an operating room. It uses a scope called a laryngoscope placed in the back of your throat. This procedure allows the doctor to see deeper in the throat and to take a tissue sample for a biopsy. The purpose of direct laryngoscopy is to identify the primary (main) tumor and determine if it is resectable (can be removed with surgery).

Esophagoscopy

In an esophagoscopy, a device is guided down the throat into the esophagus. It is performed under anesthesia in an operating room. This allows the doctor to examine your esophagus (swallowing tube) for abnormal growths.

Bronchoscopy

During a bronchoscopy, a device is inserted through the nose or mouth to examine the inside of your airway, including the trachea and bronchi. Bronchoscopy may be used to detect cancer or to perform some treatment procedures. It is done under anesthesia to make you more comfortable.

Panendoscopy

During a panendoscopy, different types of endoscopes are passed down the mouth or nose to do a laryngoscopy, pharyngoscopy, esophagoscopy, or bronchoscopy. This allows a doctor to thoroughly examine the mouth, oropharynx, larynx (voice box), esophagus (tube leading to the stomach), and trachea (windpipe) and bronchi (breathing passages in the lungs). It is performed under anesthesia to make you more comfortable.

This procedure might be done to look for other tumors if it is unclear where the cancer started, or if the lymph nodes in the bottom part of the neck seem abnormal. A biopsy of any tumors or other abnormal areas might be taken. Biopsies can be done with special tools that are used through the scopes.

Create a medical binder

A medical binder or notebook is a great way to organize all of your records in one place.

- ✓ Make copies of blood tests, imaging results, and reports about your specific type of cancer. It will be helpful when getting a second opinion.
- ✓ Choose a binder that meets your needs. Consider a zipper pocket to include a pen, small calendar, and insurance cards.
- ✓ Create folders for insurance forms, test types (ie, blood, imaging, pathology, radiology, genetics), treatments, and procedures. Organize items in the folder by date.
- ✓ Use online patient portals to view your test results and other records. Download or print the records to add to your binder.
- ✓ Add a section for questions and to take notes.

Bring your medical binder to appointments. You never know when you might need it!

Biopsy

A biopsy removes a sample of tissue or fluid. Samples removed during a biopsy or surgery will be sent to a pathologist, an expert in examining cells using a microscope (called cytology) to confirm the presence of cancer. The pathologist will determine the cancer subtype called tumor histology.

A fine-needle aspiration (FNA), fine-needle biopsy (FNB), and core needle biopsy (CNB) use needles of different sizes to remove a sample of tumor or lymph node. An ultrasound (US) or CT scan might be used to guide a lymph node biopsy.

Biopsy of metastasis

Metastasis is the spread of cancer to an area of the body such as lymph nodes or lung. A biopsy of the metastasis may be needed to confirm the presence of cancer. If there is more than one metastasis, each site may be biopsied. The type of biopsy used depends on the location of the suspected metastases and other factors.

Biomarker testing

Biomarker tumor testing includes tests of genes or their products (proteins). It identifies the presence or absence of mutations and certain proteins that might suggest treatment. This information is used to choose the best treatment for you. It is sometimes called molecular testing or tumor profiling, tumor sequencing, gene expression profiling, or genomic testing.

Inside our cells are deoxyribonucleic acid (DNA) molecules. These molecules are tightly packaged into what is called a chromosome. Chromosomes contain most of the genetic information in a cell. Normal human cells contain 23 pairs of chromosomes for a total of 46 chromosomes. Each chromosome contains thousands of genes. Genes are coded instructions for the proteins your cells make. Most genes contain information about a specific protein. A mutation is when something goes wrong in the genetic code.

MSI-H/dMMR mutation

Microsatellites are short, repeated strings of DNA. When errors or defects occur, they are fixed by mismatch repair (MMR) proteins. Some cancers have DNA mutations or changes that prevent these errors from being fixed. This is called microsatellite instability (MSI) or deficient mismatch repair (dMMR). When cancer cells have more than a normal number of microsatellites, it is called MSI-H (microsatellite instability-high). This is often due to dMMR genes.

PD-L1 testing

Programmed death-ligand 1 (PD-L1) is an immune protein. If this protein is expressed on the surface of cancer cells, it can cause your immune cells to ignore the cancer and suppress the anti-tumor immune response. This is designed to activate your immune system to better fight off the cancer cells. PD-L1 expression is measured using a combined positive score (CPS), which measures the immune proteins in your tumor and your immune system. If your cancer expresses this protein and has a CPS of at least 1 percent (1%) or higher, you might have treatment that combines chemotherapy and an immune checkpoint inhibitor therapy, or have immune checkpoint inhibitor therapy by itself.

Tumor p16 (HPV) testing

HPV testing by p16 is recommended for everyone diagnosed with throat (oropharyngeal) cancer. It is used to learn more information about your cancer. Testing will be done on a biopsy of your tumor from either your throat, a lymph node, or other sites in your body if needed.

Tumor mutational burden

When there are 10 or more mutations per million base pairs of tumor DNA, it is called tumor mutational burden-high (TMB-H). Metastatic or unresectable TMB cancers are often treated using immune checkpoint inhibitors that target the proteins called programmed cell death protein 1 (PD-1) and programmed death-ligand 1 (PD-L1).

Tumor mutation testing

Tumor mutation testing or tumor genomic aberration testing uses a sample of your tumor or blood to see if the cancer cells have any specific DNA mutations. This is a different type of DNA testing than the genetic testing for mutations you may have inherited from your biological parents. In tumor mutation testing, only the tumor is tested and not the rest of your body. Some mutations can be targeted with specific therapies.

Cell-free DNA testing

Cell-free or circulating tumor DNA (ctDNA) testing uses a sample of blood to look for cancer cells or for pieces of DNA from tumor cells. Although this test is not a recommended standard and its use has not been agreed upon, many providers use it to monitor treatment response and for cancer recurrence.

Key points

- Results from imaging studies and a biopsy will determine your treatment plan. Often, information is collected over time, even as treatment begins. Online portals are a great way to access your test results. Please discuss your results with your health care provider.
- A medical history and physical exam inform your care team about your overall health. Your overall health may guide the best treatment for your cancer.
- Head and neck cancer and its treatment can affect the health of your jaw, teeth, and gums. Tell your dentist about your head and neck cancer and keep up with regular dental cleanings and checkups.
- Treatment can affect fertility. Talk to your care team about your concerns and if you are planning a pregnancy.
- Imaging tests take pictures of the inside of your body.
- An exam of the throat (pharynx) may sometimes involve the use of a thin, tube-shaped tool called a scope that is inserted into the mouth or nose.
- A biopsy removes a sample of tissue or fluid for testing.
- A sample of your tumor may be tested to look for specific DNA (deoxyribonucleic acid) mutations, protein levels, or other molecular features. Some mutations and proteins can be targeted with specific therapies.
- HPV testing by p16 is recommended for everyone diagnosed with throat (oropharyngeal) cancer.

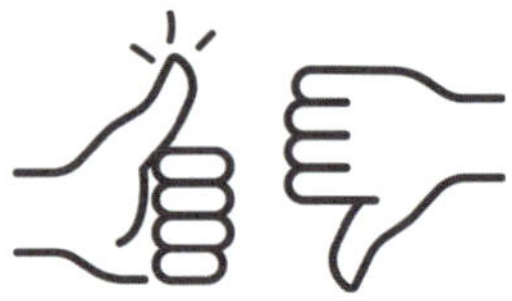

Let us know what you think!

Please take a moment to complete an online survey about the NCCN Guidelines for Patients.

NCCN.org/patients/response

3

Throat cancer staging

Cancer staging is used to reflect prognosis and to guide treatment decisions. It describes the size and location of the tumor and if cancer has spread to lymph nodes or other parts of the body. Testing for p16 (HPV) is an important part of staging. This chapter explains throat cancer stages.

How throat cancer is staged

A cancer stage is a way to describe the extent of the cancer at the time you are first diagnosed. The American Joint Committee on Cancer (AJCC) created a staging system to determine how much cancer is in your body, where it is located, and what subtype you have. This is called staging. Cancer staging is not the same for all cancer types and locations.

Based on testing, your cancer will be assigned a stage. Staging helps to predict prognosis and is needed to make treatment decisions. A prognosis is the course your cancer will likely take. AJCC is just one type of staging system.

Information gathered during staging:

- **The extent (size) of the tumor (T):** How large is the cancer? Has it grown into nearby areas?
- **The spread to nearby lymph nodes (N):** Has the cancer spread to nearby lymph nodes? If so, how many? Where?
- **The spread (metastasis) to distant sites (M):** Has the cancer spread to distant organs such as the lungs or liver?
- **Grade of the cancer (G):** How much do the cancer cells look like normal cells?
- **Biomarker testing:** Does the cancer have any genes, proteins such as p16, or mutations that might suggest treatment?

Staging is based on a combination of information to reach a final numbered stage. Often, not all information is available at the initial evaluation. More information can be gathered as treatment begins. Doctors may explain your cancer stage in different ways than described next.

Staging includes:

- **Anatomic** – based on extent of cancer as defined by tumor size (T), lymph node status (N), and distant metastasis (M).
- **Prognostic** – includes anatomic TNM plus tumor grade. The prognostic stage also includes the assumption that you are treated with the standard-of-care approaches.

Prognostic stages are divided into clinical and pathologic. Cancer staging is often done twice, before and after surgery. Staging after surgery provides more specific and accurate details about the size of the cancer and lymph node status.

Clinical stage

Clinical stage (c) is the rating given before any treatment. It is based on a physical exam, biopsy, and imaging tests. An example might look like cN2 or cM1. In throat cancer, the clinical (before surgery) stage is based on imaging results. These tests are done before any treatment as part of an initial diagnosis. Surgery is needed to know exactly how much cancer is in the body.

Pathologic stage

Pathologic stage (p) or surgical stage is determined by examining tissue removed during surgery. An example might be pN2. If you are given a cancer drug therapy before surgery, then the stage might add a "y" and look like ypT3. The pathologic (after surgery) stage is based on information gained after surgery to remove all or part of the tumor and nearby lymph nodes. This gives a more accurate picture of how far the cancer has spread and is used to determine your treatment options after surgery. The removal of tumor tissue and nearby lymph nodes is an important part of pathologic staging.

Lymph nodes in the head and neck

There are over 300 lymph nodes in the head and neck. Most throat tumors spread to nearby lymph nodes.

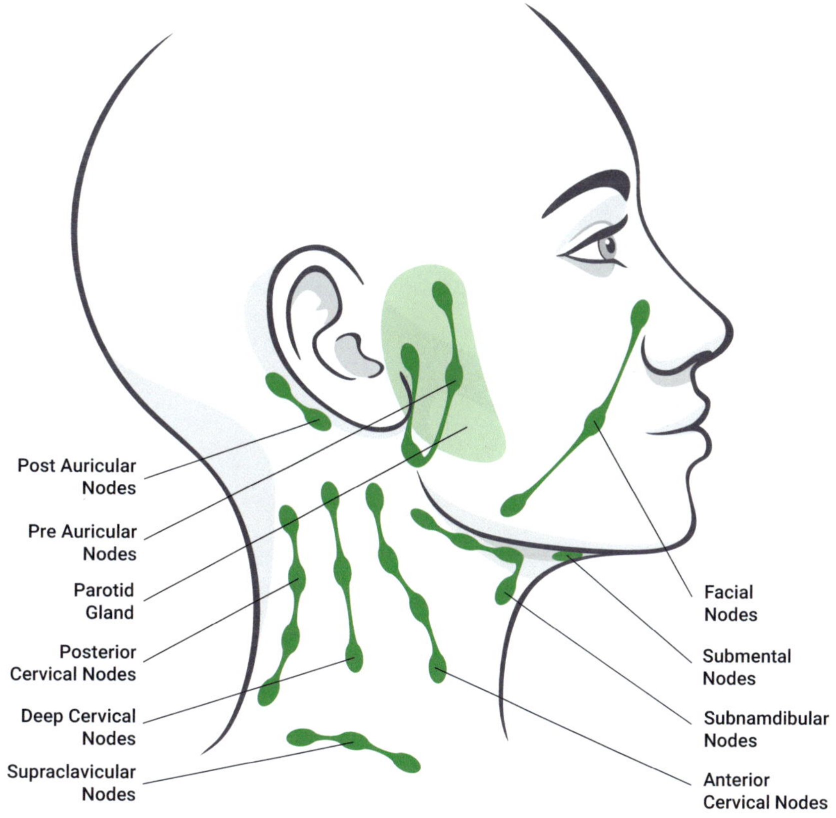

TNM scores

The tumor, node, metastasis (TNM) system is used to stage throat cancer. In this system, the letters T, N, and M describe different areas of cancer growth. Based on imaging and pathology results, a score or number is assigned to each letter. The higher the number, the larger the tumor or the more the cancer has spread. These scores will be combined to assign the cancer a stage. A TNM example might look like this: T1N0M0 or T1, N0, M0.

- **T (tumor) –** Depth and size of the main (primary) tumor
- **N (node) –** If cancer has spread to nearby (regional) lymph nodes
- **M (metastasis) –** If cancer has spread to distant parts of the body or metastasized

Throat cancer stages are based on if the cancer is p16-positive (p16+) or p16-negative (p16-). A p16+ cancer is one that is HPV-related (HPV-mediated).

Numbered stages

Numbered stages are based on TNM scores. Stages range from stage 0 to stage 4, with 4 being the most advanced. They might be written as stage 0, stage I, stage II, stage III, and stage IV.

Other terms might be used instead of numbered cancer stages.

- **Resectable –** Tumor can be removed completely with surgery.
- **Unresectable –** Tumor cannot be removed completely with surgery. The tumor might involve nearby veins and arteries or other structures making it unsafe to remove.
- **Locoregional or locally advanced –** This refers to a tumor that has spread to tissue, organs, or lymph nodes in the head and neck.
- **Moderately or very advanced disease –** Cancer that has spread to parts of the neck such as the base of the skull, larynx, pharynx, bones and muscles behind the nasal cavity, jaw, and roof of the mouth. It might include cancer in the carotid artery.
- **Metastatic –** Cancer that has spread to other parts of the body, including lung and distant lymph nodes. This might be referred to as very advanced disease. Not all stage 4 cancers are metastatic.

p16- (HPV-) cancer stages

p16- throat cancer starts in the oropharynx and is not caused by human papillomavirus (HPV). The following TNM staging information is used for squamous cell carcinoma that tested negative for p16 or was not tested. For p16- (HPV-) cancer stages, **see Guide 2**.

T = Tumor

A tumor can grow into nearby structures. Head and neck tumors are measured in centimeters (cm). A baseball is 7 cm, a golf ball is 4 cm, and a pea is 1 cm.

- **Tis** – Carcinoma in situ
- **T1** – Tumor is 2 cm or smaller
- **T2** – Tumor is between 2 and 4 cm
- **T3** – Tumor is larger than 4 cm or has grown in to the epiglottis flap that closes the airway to the trachea)
- **T4a** – Moderately advanced local disease. Tumor invades the larynx, extrinsic muscle of tongue, medial pterygoid, hard palate, or mandible.
- **T4b** – Very advanced local disease. Tumor invades lateral pterygoid muscle, pterygoid plates, lateral nasopharynx, or skull base or encases carotid artery.

Guide 2
p16- cancer stages

Stage 0	• Tis, N0, M0
Stage 1	• T1, N0, M0
Stage 2	• T2, N0, M0
Stage 3	• T3, N0, M0 • T1 or T2 or T3, N1, M0
Stage 4A	• T1 or T2 or T3, N2, M0 • T4a, N1 or N1 or N2, M0
Stage 4B	• T4b, Any N, M0 • Any T, N3, M0
Stage 4C	• Any T, Any N, M1

N = Regional lymph node

The head and neck contain a network of more than 300 nodes. They are bound together with muscles nerves, and blood and lymph vessels. Cancer can spread from these areas in to lymph nodes. When cancer has grown outside the lymph node it is referred to as extranodal extension or extranodal extension-positive (ENE+).

- **N0** – No regional lymph node metastasis is found
- **N1** – Metastasis of 3 cm or smaller is found inside 1 lymph node
- **N2** – Metastasis of 3 to 6 cm is found inside 1 or more lymph nodes
- **N3** – Metastasis of larger than 6 cm is found inside lymph node (ENE-) or metastasis of any size is found that has grown outside of the lymph node (ENE+).

"If you feel something different around your neck, glands, tongue, or mouth area, please don't wait! Go see an ear, nose, and throat (ENT) doctor."

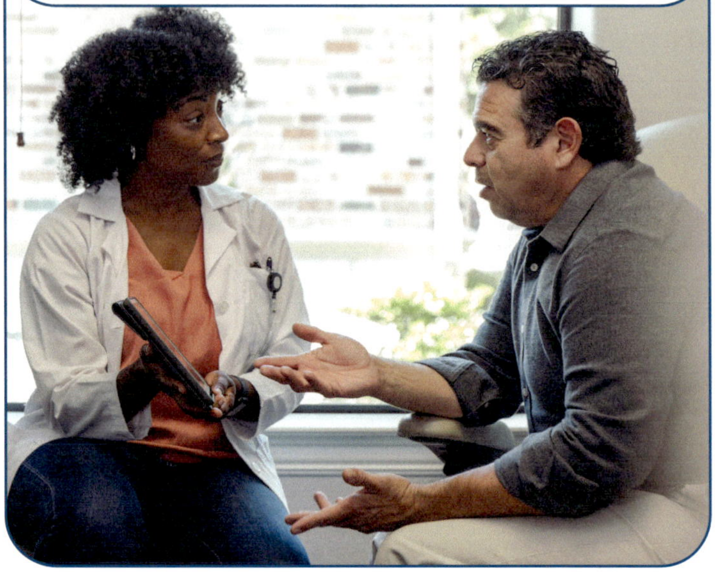

M = Metastasis

Cancer that has spread via the bloodstream to distant parts of the body is shown as M1. The most common site for metastasis is the lungs.

Grade

Grade describes how abnormal the tumor cells look under a microscope (called histology). Higher-grade cancers tend to grow and spread faster than lower-grade cancers. GX means the grade can't be determined, followed by G1, G2, G3, and G4. G4 is the highest grade for p16- (HPV-) throat cancer.

p16+ (HPV+) cancer stages

p16+ throat cancer starts in the oropharynx and is caused by human papillomavirus (HPV). For p16+ (HPV+) cancer stages, **see Guides 3 and 4**.

If squamous cell cancer is detected in a lymph node(s) in your neck, but no primary (main) tumor is found (T0) in your throat (base of tongue or tonsil), then you might have a cancer of unknown primary location. The cancer from a lymph node biopsy will be tested for p16. If cancer is p16+, then your tumor will be tested for HPV. If positive for HPV (p16+/HPV+), then you will be treated the same as those who have HPV+ primary cancers that arise in the tonsils or base of tongue. If negative for HPV (p16+/HPV-), you do not have a cancer that started in your base of tongue or tonsils. You may have a primary skin cancer that will be treated differently.

T = Tumor

A tumor can grow into nearby structures. Head and neck tumors are measured in centimeters (cm). A baseball is 7 cm, a golf ball is 4 cm, and a pea is 1 cm.

- **T0** – No tumor is found
- **T1** – Tumor is 2 cm or smaller
- **T2** – Tumor is between 2 and 4 cm
- **T3** – Tumor is larger than 4 cm or has grown into the epiglottis flap that closes the airway to the trachea
- **T4** – Moderately advanced local disease. Tumor invades the larynx, extrinsic muscle of the tongue, medial pterygoid, hard palate, or mandible or beyond.

Guide 3
p16+ before surgery cancer stages

Stage 1	• T0 or T1 or T2, N0 or N1, M0
Stage 2	• T0 or T1 or T2, N0 or N1, M0 • T3, N0 or N1 or N2, M0
Stage 3	• T0 or T1 or T2 or T3, N3, M0 • T4, N0 or N1 or N2 or N3, M0
Stage 4	• Any T, Any N, M1

Guide 4
p16+ after surgery cancer stages

Stage 1	• T0 or T1 or T2, N0 or N1, M0
Stage 2	• T0 or T1 or T2, N0 or N1, M0 • T3 or T4, N0 or N1, M0
Stage 3	• T3 or T4, N2, M0
Stage 4	• Any T, Any N, M1

N = Regional lymph node

The removal of lymph nodes is called lymph node or nodal dissection. Lymph node staging before lymph node dissection is called clinical (c) staging and is shown as cN. Staging after surgery is called pathologic (p) and is shown as pN in a pathology report.

Clinical N

- **N0** – No regional lymph node metastasis is found
- **N1** – One or more lymph nodes with metastasis are found on the same side (ipsilateral) as the tumor, none larger than 6 cm
- **N2** – Lymph nodes with metastasis are found on the opposite side (contralateral) as the tumor or on both sides (bilateral), none larger than 6 cm
- **N3** – Lymph node(s) larger than 6 cm

Pathologic N

- **pN0** – No regional lymph node metastasis is found
- **pN1** – Metastasis is found in 4 or fewer lymph nodes
- **pN2** – Metastasis is found in more than 4 lymph nodes

M = Metastasis

Cancer that has spread through the bloodstream to distant parts of the body is shown as M1. The most common site for metastasis is the lungs.

Grade

No grading system exists for p16+ (HPV+) throat cancer.

Head and neck tumors are measured in centimeters: A baseball is 7 cm, a golf ball is 4 cm, and a pea is 1 cm.

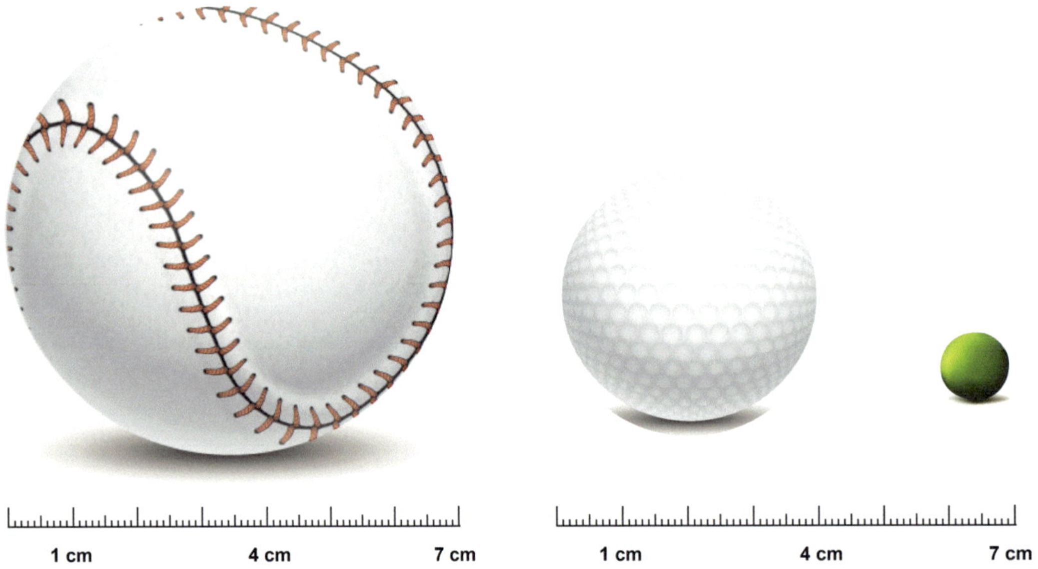

Key points

- A cancer stage helps to predict the likely course your cancer will take, called a prognosis. It describes the size and location of the tumor and if cancer has spread to lymph nodes, organs, or other parts of the body. Cancer staging is not the same for all cancer types and locations.
- Staging is used to make treatment decisions.
- In head and neck cancer, tumor testing for p16 (HPV) is an important part of staging.
- Tumors that test positive for p16 (p16+) are staged and treated differently than tumors that test negative for p16 (p16-).
- The head and neck contain a network of more than 300 nodes. They are bound together with muscles, nerves, and blood and lymph vessels. Cancer can spread from these areas into lymph nodes.
- Most throat tumors can spread, usually to nearby cervical (neck) lymph nodes.
- When cancer has grown outside the lymph node it is called extranodal extension (ENE+). When cancer has not grown outside of the lymph node it is shown as ENE-.
- Not all stage 4 cancers that have spread through the blood are metastatic and some can be cured.

We want your feedback!

Our goal is to provide helpful and easy-to-understand information on cancer.

Take our survey to let us know what we got right and what we could do better.

NCCN.org/patients/feedback

4
Treating throat cancer

Treatment decisions should include you and a multidisciplinary team of experts. This chapter describes treatment options and what to expect. Together, you and your care team will choose a treatment plan that is best for you.

Care team

Those with head and cancer should seek treatment at experienced cancer centers.

Treating cancer takes a team approach. Treatment decisions should involve a multidisciplinary team (MDT). An MDT is a team of health care and psychosocial care professionals from different professional backgrounds who have knowledge (expertise) and experience in your type of cancer. This team is united in the planning and implementation of your treatment. Ask who will coordinate your care.

Some members of your care team will be with you throughout cancer treatment, while others will only be there for parts of it. Get to know your care team and help them get to know you.

Depending on your diagnosis, your team might include the following specialists:

- **An otolaryngologist, head and neck surgeon, or surgical oncologist** can perform operations to remove cancer.
- **Oncologists** specialize in diagnosing and treating cancer. Types of oncologists include medical, radiation, and surgical oncologists.
- **Oncology nurses** provide your hands-on care, like giving systemic therapy, managing your care, answering questions, and helping you cope with side effects.
- **Oncology pharmacists** are experts in knowing how to use medicines to treat cancer and to manage symptoms and side effects.
- **Palliative care specialists** concentrate on preventing and alleviating suffering and improving quality of life.
- **Radiation therapists** provide your hands-on delivery of radiotherapy treatments.
- **Nutritionists and dietitians** can provide guidance on what foods are most suitable for your condition.
- **An occupational therapist** helps people with the tasks of daily living.
- **A physical therapist** helps people move with greater comfort and ease.
- **A certified lymphedema therapist** gives a type of massage called manual lymph drainage.
- **Speech-language and swallowing therapists** help people who have trouble speaking or swallowing.

- **Psychologists and psychiatrists** are mental health experts who can help manage issues such as depression, anxiety, or other mental health conditions that can affect how you think and feel.
- **Social workers** help people solve and cope with problems in their everyday lives. Clinical social workers also diagnose and treat mental, behavioral, and emotional conditions. The anxiety a person feels when diagnosed with cancer might be managed by a social worker in some cancer centers. They, or other designated professionals, can help navigate the complexities of financial and insurance stresses.
- **Spiritual care specialists** identify and support those with spiritual distress or unmet spiritual needs.
- **Smoking cessation specialists** can provide medication and counseling for those who would like to stop using tobacco or nicotine products.
- **A research team** helps to collect research data and coordinate care if you are in a clinical trial. Clinical trials help bring new therapies to patients and advance the treatment for everyone. Consider asking your care team about access to clinical trials.

You know your body better than anyone

Help your health care team members understand:

- How you feel
- What you need
- What is working and what is not

Keep a list of names and contact information for each member of your team. This will make it easier for you and anyone involved in your care to know whom to contact with questions or concerns.

Get to know your care team and help them get to know you.

Surgery

Surgery is an operation or procedure to remove cancer from the body. When preparing for surgery, you should seek the opinion of an experienced otolaryngologist, head and neck surgeon, or surgical oncologist with expertise in head and neck cancer. The surgeon should be an expert in performing your type of surgery. Hospitals that perform many surgeries often have better results. You can ask for a referral to a hospital or cancer center that has experience in treating your type of cancer.

The removal of the cancer through surgery can be accomplished in different ways depending on the specific circumstances, such as the size and location of the tumor, whether there is cancer in any surrounding organs and tissues, and your unique anatomy. Surgery is based on the safest and best way to remove cancer. Transoral robotic surgery (TORS) is often offered to those with p16+ cancers who are surgical candidates. TORS is a minimally invasive, robotic surgery technique that removes benign and malignant tumors of the mouth and throat.

When planning for surgery, you should ask how your breathing, swallowing, speaking, chewing, and appearance might be affected. Sometimes nerves might need to be cut and sewn back together or removed as part of cancer surgery. Lymph nodes are often removed. This is the time to ask how your neck and face might look after surgery and your options about facial reconstruction surgery.

Everyone with head and neck cancer should meet with an otolaryngologist, head and neck surgeon, or surgical oncologist who is an expert in head and neck cancer before starting treatment.

Goal of surgery

The goal of surgery is to remove all of the cancer and keep your ability to function, such as chew, swallow, breathe, and speak. During surgery, the tumor is removed along with a rim of normal-looking tissue around its edge called the surgical margin. The surgical margin may look normal but cancerous cells may be found when viewed under a microscope by a pathologist. A clear or negative margin (R0) is when no cancer cells are found in the tissue around the edge of the tumor. In a positive margin, cancer cells are found in normal-looking tissue around the tumor. Your surgeon will look carefully for cancer not only along the surgical margin, but in other nearby areas. Despite best efforts, it is not always possible to find all of the cancer. Sometimes, surgeons can't safely remove the tumor with a cancer-free margin. Surgery includes removal of lymph nodes. You may have more than one surgery.

After surgery, you may receive treatment such as radiation or chemotherapy with radiation to kill any remaining cancer cells.

Tumor resection

Surgery to remove the entire tumor is called tumor resection. Sometimes, the whole tumor cannot be removed. It depends on the tumor location, what structures are involved, how close it is to vital organs, and how function (such as swallowing and speaking) will be affected. The removal of lymph nodes is part of tumor resection.

Neck lymph nodes

There are hundreds of lymph nodes throughout your body. They work as filters to help fight infection and remove harmful things from your body. Lymph is a clear fluid that gives cells water and food. It also helps to fight germs. Lymph drains from lymph tissue and travels through lymphatic vessels into lymph nodes.

The head and neck contain a network of more than 300 nodes. They are bound together with muscles, nerves, and blood and lymph vessels. Cancer can spread into these areas and nearby lymph nodes. Throat cancer often spreads to lymph nodes or lymph node groups called chains.

There are 10 (X) levels or groups of lymph nodes in the head and neck. Cervical lymph nodes are found only in the neck. The 6 (VI) levels for neck lymph node groups are described below. Lymph nodes from levels 2, 3, and 5 are at the greatest risk for throat cancer metastasis.

- **Level 1 (I)** – Submental and Submandibular Group (under the jaw line)
  - 1A – Submental nodes
  - 1B – Submandibular nodes
  - 1A and 1B are separated by the front part of a neck muscle (digastric muscle)
- **Level 2 (II)** – Upper Jugular Group (the upper neck)
  - 2A and 2B are separated by the spinal accessory nerve
- **Level 3 (III)** – Middle Jugular Group (the middle neck)
- **Level 4 (IV)** – Lower Jugular Group (the lower neck)
- **Level 5 (V)** – Posterior Triangle Group (the back portion of the neck)
  - 5A superior half (toward the head)
  - 5B inferior half (away from the head)
- **6 (VI)** – Central (Anterior) Compartment Group (in front of the windpipe)
  - Cricoid is the ring-shaped cartilage of the larynx. A "U" or "L" may be used for any N category to indicate metastasis above the lower border of the cricoid (U) or below the lower border of the cricoid (L) in this group.

Lymph node surgery

The removal of lymph nodes or groups of lymph nodes is called lymph node or nodal dissection. It might be referred to as cervical lymphadenectomy or neck dissection and is part of tumor resection surgery. Lymph nodes will be removed on the side of the neck where the main (primary) tumor is found. When the tumor is near the center of the neck (midline), then lymph nodes from both sides will be removed. The type of neck dissection is based on tumor location and information gathered in the pre-surgery (clinical) staging.

There are 3 types of cervical (neck) lymph node dissections:

- **Selective neck dissection (SND)** removes some of the regional lymph nodes where the cancer is likely to travel.
- **Comprehensive neck dissection** removes all lymph nodes in a group or level.
- **Radical neck dissection** removes all lymph nodes, and may require removing veins, arteries, nerves, or muscle next to the nodes.

Neck lymph node groups or levels

Cervical lymph nodes are found only in the neck. The 6 (VI) levels for neck lymph node groups are pictured on the right. Lymph nodes from levels 2, 3, and 5 are at the greatest risk for throat cancer metastasis.

Lymph Node Groups of the Neck

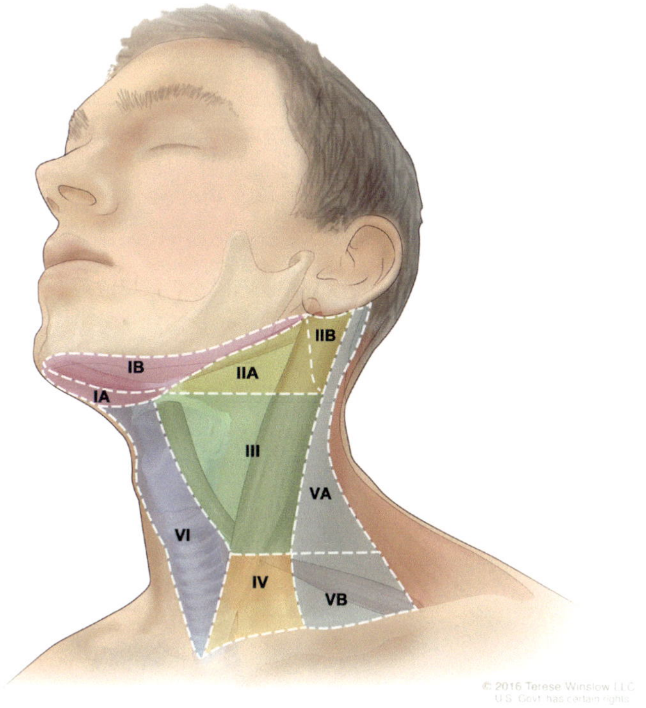

Systemic therapy

Systemic therapy works throughout the body. Types include chemotherapy, targeted therapy, and immunotherapy. Systemic therapy might be used alone or with other therapies. Goals of systemic therapy may be curative or palliative and should be discussed before starting treatment. The choice of systemic therapy will be based on your individual needs. Your wishes about treatment are important. Make your wishes known.

- When systemic therapy is given before surgery or chemoradiation, it is called **neoadjuvant or induction therapy.**
- When systemic therapy, chemoradiation, or radiation therapy is given after surgery, it is called **adjuvant or postoperative therapy.**
- When systemic therapy is given for advanced or metastatic disease, it may be called **palliative therapy**

For systemic therapy examples, **see Guide 5**.

Chemotherapy

Chemotherapy kills fast-dividing cells throughout the body, including cancer cells and some normal cells. Sometimes, chemotherapy drugs may be used in combination. This is called multiagent chemotherapy. Chemotherapy might be followed by radiation therapy or chemoradiation.

Chemoradiation

Treatment that combines chemotherapy with radiation therapy is called chemoradiation. Chemotherapy may improve how well radiation works, and that is why they are sometimes used together. For locally advanced disease, the drug cisplatin is preferred with radiation. Chemoradiation may be used to control symptoms caused by a tumor.

Guide 5
Systemic therapy examples

Chemotherapy examples	• Carboplatin • Cisplatin • Docetaxel (Taxotere) • 5-fluorouracil (5-FU)	• Gemcitabine • Methotrexate • Paclitaxel (Taxol) • Pemetrexed (Alimta)
Targeted therapy examples	• Afatinib (Gilotrif) • Cetuximab (Erbitux)	
Immunotherapy examples	• Ipilimumab (Yervoy) • Nivolumab (Opdivo) • Pembrolizumab (Keytruda)	

Targeted therapy

Targeted therapy focuses on specific or unique features of cancer cells. Targeted therapies seek out how cancer cells grow, divide, and move in the body. These drugs stop or inhibit the action of molecules that help cancer cells grow and/or survive. If your tumor has certain mutations, targeted therapy might be used. If your tumor has a high number of mutations, immunotherapy might be given.

Immunotherapy

Immunotherapy is a type of systemic treatment that tries to re-activate the immune system against tumor cells. The immune system has many on and off switches. Tumors take advantage of "off switches." Two leading off switches are programmed cell death protein 1 (PD-1) and cytotoxic T-lymphocyte–associated antigen 4 (CTLA-4). Immunotherapy can be given alone or with other types of treatment.

For more information, see NCCN Guidelines for Patients: Immunotherapy Side Effects, available at NCCN.org/patientguidelines and on the NCCN Patient Guides for Cancer app.

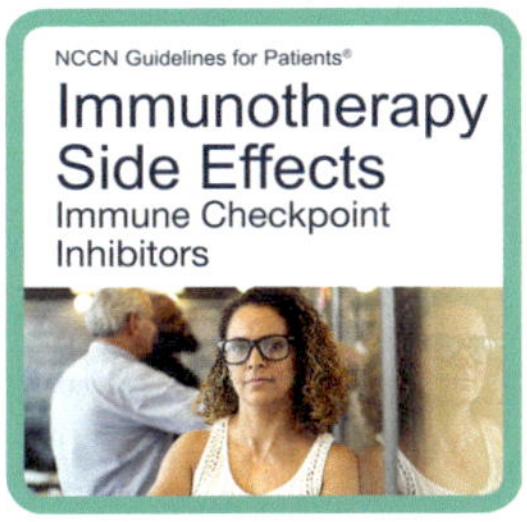

Standard of care is the best-known way to treat a particular disease based on past clinical trials. There may be more than one treatment regimen that is considered standard of care. Ask your care team what treatment options are available and if a clinical trial might be right for you.

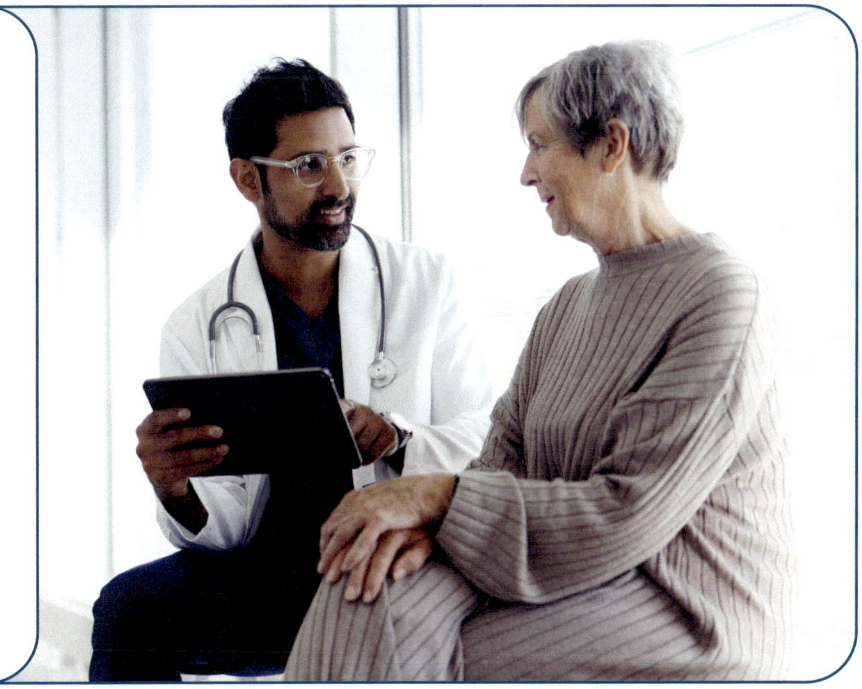

Radiation therapy

Radiation therapy (RT) uses high-energy radiation from x-rays, photons, electrons, and other sources to kill cancer cells and shrink tumors. RT may be used as main treatment to cure cancer (curative treatment), or as supportive care along with surgery or drug therapy, or for palliative care to help ease pain or discomfort caused by advanced cancer. Most types of radiation include short treatment sessions that are given once daily over a few days to weeks. Each daily treatment takes 10 to 20 minutes. RT treatment can cause a narrowing (stenosis) of the carotid artery, and an RT dose to the carotid artery can increase your risk for stroke. Ask your care team which radiation option(s) are best for your situation, if RT will be combined with chemotherapy, and what side effects to expect.

Panoramic dental x-ray is part of a pre-radiation therapy dental evaluation. It is needed to check the health of your jaw and teeth to see if you need any dental work before starting radiation therapy. It is important to tell your dentist about your head and neck cancer and to have regular dental cleanings and checkups.

Radiation therapy

External beam radiation therapy (EBRT) uses a machine outside the body to aim radiation at the tumor(s) or areas of the body.

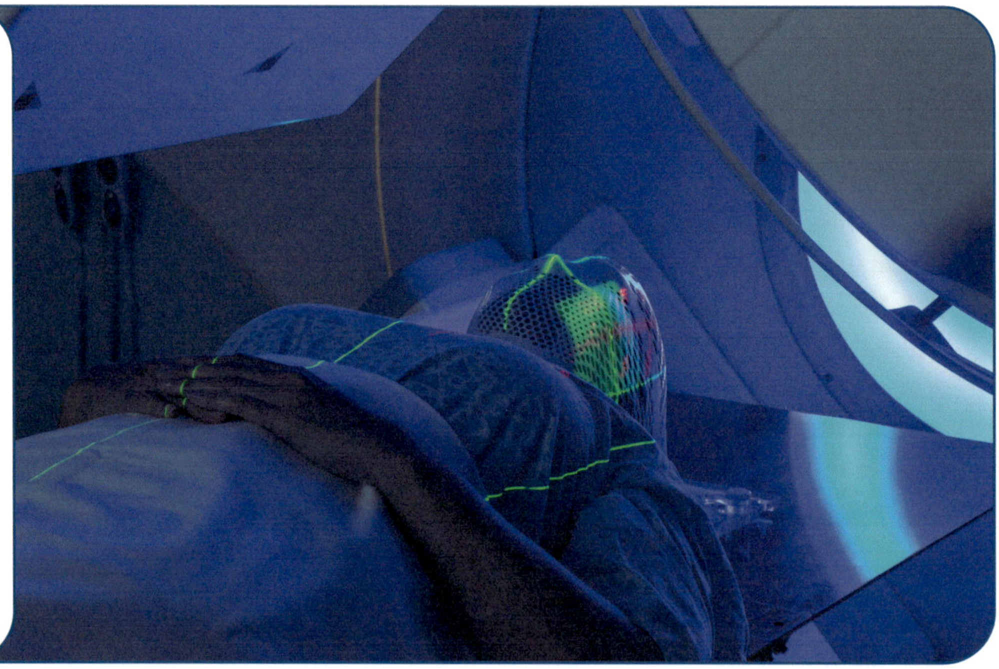

EBRT

External beam radiation therapy (EBRT) uses a machine outside the body to aim radiation at the tumor(s) or areas of the body.

Common types of EBRT that may be used to treat your cancer include the following:

- **Three-dimensional conformal radiation therapy (3D-CRT)** uses computer software and CT images to aim beams that match the shape of the tumor.
- **Intensity-modulated radiation therapy (IMRT)** uses small beams of different strengths to match the shape of the tumor. This limits the amount of radiation to normal tissue.
- **Stereotactic body radiation therapy (SBRT)** uses high-energy proton or photon beams to kill or ablate the tumor. SBRT is very precise, which reduces the chance of damage to nearby tissues.
- **Proton beam therapy (PBT)** uses proton beams to kill or ablate the tumor. It is used as a second radiation option after another type of radiation was used before.

Either IMRT (preferred) or 3D-CRT is often recommended for throat cancer to minimize radiation dose to critical structures.

Clinical trials

A clinical trial is a type of medical research study. After being developed and tested in a laboratory, potential new ways of treating cancer need to be studied in people. If found to be safe and effective in a clinical trial, a drug, device, or treatment approach may be approved by the U.S. Food and Drug Administration (FDA).

Everyone with cancer should carefully consider all of the treatment options available for their cancer type, including standard treatments and clinical trials. Talk to your doctor about whether a clinical trial may make sense for you.

Phases

Most cancer clinical trials focus on treatment. Treatment trials are done in phases.

- **Phase I trials** study the dose, safety, and side effects of an investigational drug or treatment approach. They also look for early signs that the drug or approach is helpful.
- **Phase II trials** study how well the drug or approach works against a specific type of cancer.
- **Phase III trials** test the drug or approach against a standard treatment. If the results are good, it may be approved by the FDA.
- **Phase IV trials** study the long-term safety and benefit of an FDA-approved treatment.

Who can enroll?

Every clinical trial has rules for joining, called eligibility criteria. The rules may be about age, cancer type and stage, treatment history, lab tests, or general health. These requirements ensure that participants are alike in specific ways and that the trial is as safe as possible for the participants.

Informed consent

Clinical trials are managed by a group of experts called a research team. The research team will review the study with you in detail, including its purpose and the risks and benefits of joining. All of this information is also provided in an informed consent form. Read the form carefully and ask questions before signing it. Take time to discuss with family, friends, or others whom you trust. Keep in mind that you can leave and seek treatment outside of the clinical trial at any time.

Start the conversation

Don't wait for your doctor to bring up clinical trials. Start the conversation and learn about all of your treatment options. If you find a study that you may be eligible for, ask your treatment team if you meet the requirements. If you have already started standard treatment, then you may not be eligible for certain clinical trials. Try not to be discouraged if you cannot join. New clinical trials are always becoming available.

Frequently asked questions

There are many myths and misconceptions surrounding clinical trials. The possible benefits and risks are not well understood by many with cancer.

Will I get a placebo?
Placebos (inactive versions of real medicines) are almost never used alone in cancer clinical trials. It is common to receive either a placebo with a standard treatment, or a new drug with a standard treatment. You will be informed, verbally and in writing, if a placebo is part of a clinical trial before you enroll.

Do I have to pay to be in a clinical trial?
It depends on the study, your health insurance, and the state in which you live. In general, procedures, drugs, or tests that are considered standard of care will be billed to you or your insurance, whereas those considered research are covered by the trial sponsor. Your treatment team and the research team can help determine if you are responsible for any costs.

Supportive care

Supportive care will be specific to your needs. Supportive care is health care given to prevent, reduce, and relieve suffering, and to improve quality of life. Supportive care might include pain relief, palliative care, emotional or spiritual support, financial aid, or family counseling. Tell your care team how you are feeling and about any side effects so they can be managed. Supportive care, best supportive care, and palliative care often mean the same thing.

It is very important to take care of yourself by eating well, drinking plenty of fluids, exercising, and doing things that make you feel energized. Strength is needed to sustain you during treatment.

Side effects

All cancer treatments can cause unwanted health issues called side effects. Side effects depend on many factors. These factors include the drug type and dose, length of treatment, and the person. Some side effects may be harmful to your health. Others may just be unpleasant. Treatment can cause several side effects. Some are very serious.

Ask for a complete list of side effects of your treatments. Also, tell your treatment team about any new or worsening symptoms. There may be ways to help you feel better. There are also ways to prevent some side effects. You will be monitored closely for side effects.

It is important to tell your care team about all side effects so they can be managed.

Late effects

Late effects are side effects that occur months or years after a disease is diagnosed or after treatment has ended. Late effects may be caused by cancer or cancer treatment. They may include physical, mental, and social problems, and second cancers (caused by the treatment itself). The sooner late effects are treated the better. Ask your care team about what late effects could occur. This will help you know what to look for.

Survivorship

A person is a cancer survivor from the time of diagnosis until the end of life. When treatment leads to remission (or no evidence of disease), you will need follow-up or survivorship care for late effects. During survivorship care you will still have a care team, but it will look different. Seek out peer support groups, whether online or in person.

Side effects

Diarrhea

Diarrhea is frequent and watery bowel movements, or more bowel movements than usual. It is a common side effect of chemotherapy. Diarrhea is treated with prescription and over-the-counter (OTC) medicines, and food recommendations (like eating rice or bread). Do not take any OTC medicines without speaking to your care team first. It is not unusual for diarrhea medicines to cause constipation. Your care team will tell you how to manage diarrhea and constipation. It is important to drink lots of fluids.

Difficulty breathing

Difficulty breathing or shortness of breath (called dyspnea) is very common. How it feels and the level of discomfort is different for everyone. Non-drug therapies are recommended such as the use of handheld fans directed at the face, cooler temperatures, stress management, relaxation therapy, and emotional and psychosocial support. Depending on the cause or type of discomfort, dyspnea might be treated with systemic therapy, radiation therapy (RT), medicine, or oxygen.

Difficulty eating and loss of appetite

Sometimes side effects from surgery, cancer, or its treatment, and the stress of having cancer might cause you to feel not hungry or sick to your stomach (nauseated). You might have a sore mouth or difficulty swallowing. Healthy eating is important during treatment. It includes eating a balanced diet, eating the right amount of food, and drinking enough fluids. A registered dietitian who is an expert in nutrition and food can help. Weight loss is common in those with head and neck cancer. You might be asked to see a nutrition expert before starting treatment to help prevent severe weight loss.

Supportive care resources

More information on supportive care is available at: NCCN.org/patientguidelines and on the NCCN Patient Guides for Cancer app.

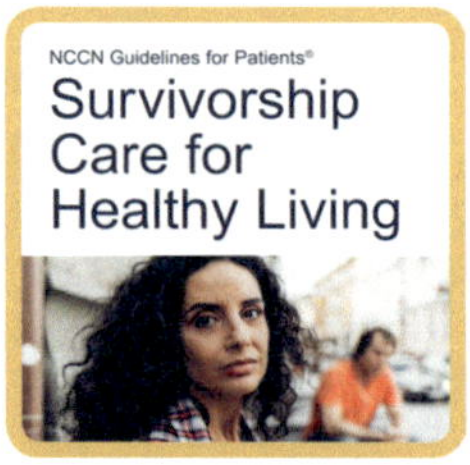

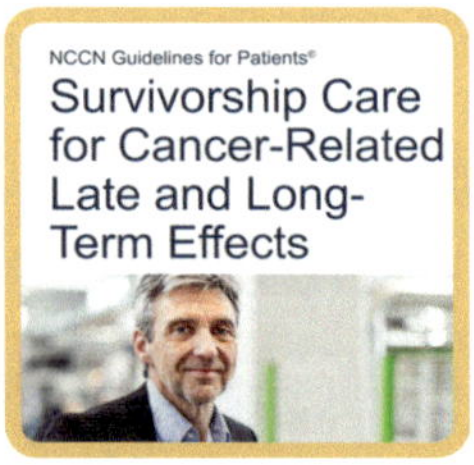

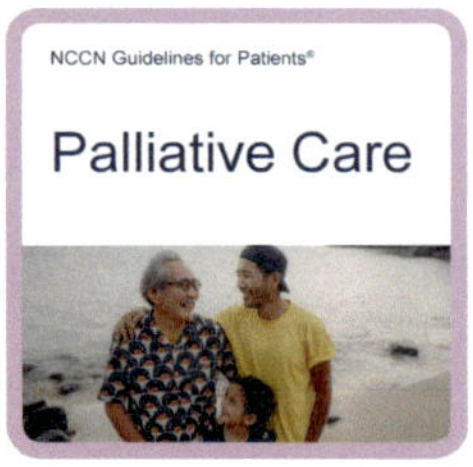

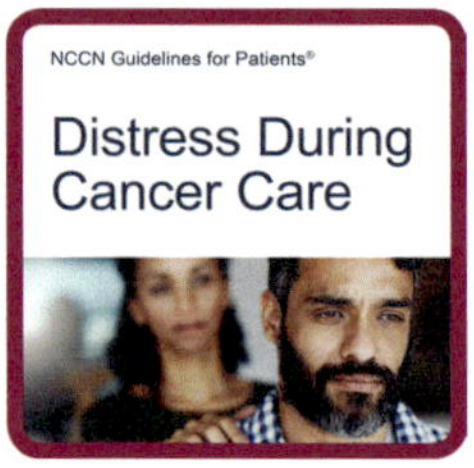

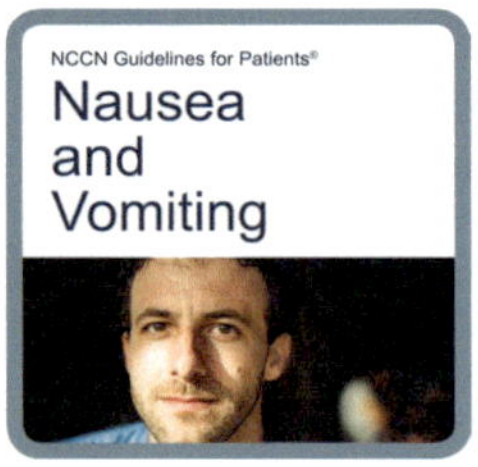

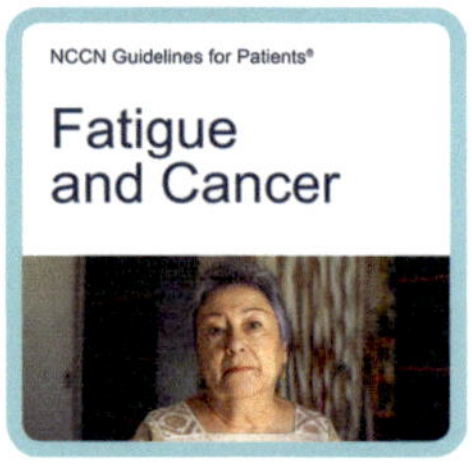

Difficulty swallowing or speaking

Difficult swallowing (dysphagia) or painful swallowing (odynophagia) can be caused by treatment. Speech-language pathologists (SLPs) can help people who have trouble swallowing or speaking as a result of surgery or radiation therapy.

Distress

Depression, anxiety, and sleeping issues are common and are a normal part of cancer diagnosis. Talk to your care team and with those whom you feel most comfortable about how you are feeling. There are services, people, and medicine that can help you. Support and counseling services are available.

Fatigue

Fatigue is extreme tiredness and inability to function due to lack of energy. Fatigue may be caused by cancer or it may be a side effect of treatment. Let your care team know how you are feeling and if fatigue is getting in the way of doing the things you enjoy. Eating a balanced diet, exercise, yoga, acupuncture, and massage therapy can help. You might be referred to a nutritionist or dietitian to help with fatigue.

Keep a pain diary

A pain diary is a written record that helps you keep track of when you have pain, how bad it is, what causes it, and what makes it better or worse. Use a pain diary to discuss your pain with your care team. You might be referred to a specialist for pain management.

Include in your pain diary:

- ✓ The time and dose of all medicines
- ✓ When pain starts and ends or lessens
- ✓ Where you feel pain
- ✓ A description of your pain. Is it throbbing, sharp, tingling, shooting, or burning? Is it constant, or does it come and go?
- ✓ Does the pain change at different times of day? When?
- ✓ Does the pain get worse before or after meals? Does certain food or drink make it better?
- ✓ Does the pain get better or worse with activity? What kind of activity?
- ✓ Does the pain keep you from falling asleep at night? Does pain wake you up in the night?
- ✓ A rating of your pain from 0 (no pain) to 10 (worst pain you have ever felt)
- ✓ Does pain get in the way of you doing the things you enjoy?

Lymphedema

Lymphedema is a condition in which lymph fluid builds up in tissues and causes swelling. It may be caused when part of the lymph system is damaged or blocked, such as during surgery to remove lymph nodes, or by radiation therapy. Cancers that block lymph vessels can also cause lymphedema. Swelling usually develops slowly over time. It may develop during treatment, or it may start years after treatment. If you have lymphedema, you may be referred to an expert in lymphedema management. The swelling may be reduced by exercise, massage, compression devices, and other means.

Nausea and vomiting

Nausea and vomiting are common side effects of treatment. You will be given medicine to prevent nausea and vomiting.

Pain

Tell your care team about any pain or discomfort. You might meet with a palliative care specialist or with a pain specialist to manage pain. Some people may benefit from palliative radiation therapy to help relieve pain. During this treatment, a radiation beam is focused on the tumor or metastasis.

Quality of life

Cancer and its treatment can affect your overall well-being or quality of life (QOL). Head and neck tumors often impact a person's ability to function such as chew, swallow, speak, and breathe. They can also impact taste, smell, hearing, how your voice sounds, or how you look. It is very important that you are well-prepared and understand how surgery or radiation therapy might cause changes to these functions and your appearance.

For more information on quality of life, see NCCN Guidelines for Patients: Palliative Care at NCCN.org/patientguidelines and on the NCCN Patient Guides for Cancer app.

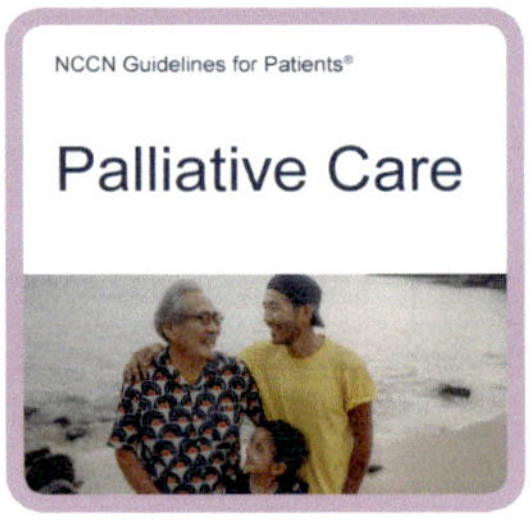

Key points

- A resectable tumor can be removed with surgery. An unresectable tumor cannot be removed with surgery because it is too close to vital organs.
- Systemic therapy works throughout the body. It includes chemotherapy, targeted therapy, and immunotherapy.
- Chemotherapy kills fast-dividing cells throughout the body, including cancer cells and some normal cells.
- Targeted therapy can block the ways cancer cells grow, divide, and move in the body.
- Immunotherapy uses your body's natural defenses to find and destroy cancer cells.
- Radiation therapy (RT) uses high-energy radiation from x-rays, gamma rays, protons, photons, and other sources to kill cancer cells and shrink tumors.
- A clinical trial is a type of research that studies a treatment to see how safe it is and how well it works.
- Supportive care is health care that relieves symptoms caused by cancer or its treatment and improves quality of life. Supportive care is always given.
- All cancer treatments can cause unwanted health issues called side effects. It is important for you to tell your care team about all your side effects so they can be managed.
- Eating a balanced diet, drinking enough fluids, exercise, and massage therapy can help manage side effects.
- Pain may be treated with medication, or radiation with or without systemic therapy. Keeping a pain diary and working with a cancer pain specialist might help you manage pain.
- Stopping smoking or vaping is essential to maximize the chance for cure and minimize side effects.

5

p16- (HPV-) cancer

A p16-negative (p16-) throat cancer is not caused by the HPV16 virus. Treatment is based on tumor location and if any lymph nodes have cancer. Together, you and your care team will choose a treatment plan that is best for you.

For throat cancer, biopsy samples are tested for the p16 protein to see if HPV infection is present. This is a key part of staging (finding out if and how much the cancer has spread) and is considered when making treatment decisions. This information can also help predict the likely course the cancer will take called a prognosis. Other factors such as your overall health are considered when making treatment decisions. Your preferences about treatment are always important. Talk to your care team and make your wishes known.

Early stage

In early-stage cancer, the tumor is 4 cm or less and cancer may be in one lymph node.

Treatment options include:

- Surgery to remove the tumor and lymph nodes (called tumor resection and neck dissection). RT or chemoradiation might follow surgery.
- Radiation therapy (RT)
- Chemoradiation, **see Guide 6.**
- Clinical trial

Guide 6
Chemoradiation examples

Preferred	• Cisplatin • Carboplatin with 5-FU
Other recommended	• Cisplatin • Carboplatin with paclitaxel
Used in some cases	• Docetaxel (if cisplatin ineligible) • 5-FU with hydroxyurea • Cetuximab • Cisplatin with 5-FU • Cisplatin with paclitaxel

Locally advanced

In locally advanced cancer, the tumor may be any size and cancer may be in 1 or more lymph nodes. The tumor might have grown into the larynx (voice box) or other nearby structures.

Treatment options include:

- Chemoradiation, **see Guide 6**.
- Surgery to remove the tumor and lymph nodes. RT or chemoradiation might follow surgery.
- Clinical trial

Follow-up care

After treatment, you will be monitored for side effects and the return of cancer called recurrence. General follow-up care includes doctor visits, blood and imaging tests, and supportive care as needed. It is important to contact your doctor right away if you notice any changes in your head or neck. For general follow-up care, **see Guide 7.**

Guide 7 **Follow-up care**
Medical history and physical exam, including complete head and neck exam: • Year 1, every 1 to 3 months • Year 2, every 2 to 6 months • Years 3 through 5, every 4 to 8 months • Over 5 years, every 12 months
Blood, spit (saliva), or urine tests to look for hormone levels made by glands in the head and neck
FDG-PET/CT at 3 months post-treatment. Other imaging tests as needed.
Dental exam for areas exposed to radiation treatment
Supportive care, as needed: • Speech, hearing, and swallowing evaluation and rehabilitation • Nutrition evaluation and rehabilitation • Ongoing screening for depression • Help to quit smoking; tobacco use and alcohol use counseling • Lymphedema evaluation and rehabilitation
Information on survivorship care and creation of a survivorship care plan within 1 year of completing treatment

Key points

- A p16-negative (p16-) throat cancer is not caused by the HPV16 virus.
- In early-stage cancer, the tumor is 4 cm or less and cancer may be in one lymph node.
- Treatment options for early-stage cancer include surgery to remove tumor and lymph nodes, radiation therapy (RT), chemoradiation, or clinical trial.
- In locally advanced cancer, the tumor may be any size and cancer may be in 1 or more lymph nodes. The tumor might have grown into the larynx (voice box) or other nearby structures.
- Treatment options for locally advanced cancer include chemoradiation, surgery to remove tumor and lymph nodes, or clinical trial.
- After completing treatment, you will have follow-up care to monitor for sides effects and changes in your health. Contact your doctor right away if you notice any changes in your head or neck.

Need help paying for medicine or treatment?

Ask your care team what options are available.

6

p16+ (HPV+) cancer

A p16-positive (p16+) throat cancer is caused by the HPV16 virus. Throat cancer linked to HPV tends to respond better to treatment than cancers that are not HPV-related. Together, you and your care team will choose a treatment plan that is best for you.

Tumor samples are tested for the p16 protein to see if HPV infection is present. This is a key part of staging (finding out if and how much the cancer has spread) and is considered when making treatment decisions. Also, there are some new blood tests that can help personalize care in HPV-positive cancers. This information can help predict the likely course the cancer will take called a prognosis.

Other factors such as your overall health are considered when making treatment decisions. Your preferences about treatment are always important. Talk to your care team and make your wishes known.

Early stage

In early-stage cancer, the tumor is 4 cm or less and cancer may be in one lymph node. If cancer is found in the lymph node, it is 3 cm or less.

Treatment options include:

- Surgery to remove the tumor and lymph nodes (called tumor resection and neck dissection). Transoral robotic surgery (TORS) is often offered to those with p16+ cancers who are surgical candidates. Radiation therapy (RT) or chemoradiation might follow surgery.

Seek out support groups at your local hospital, through social media, or from those listed in the back of this book. Look to friends, relatives, neighbors, and coworkers for social support.

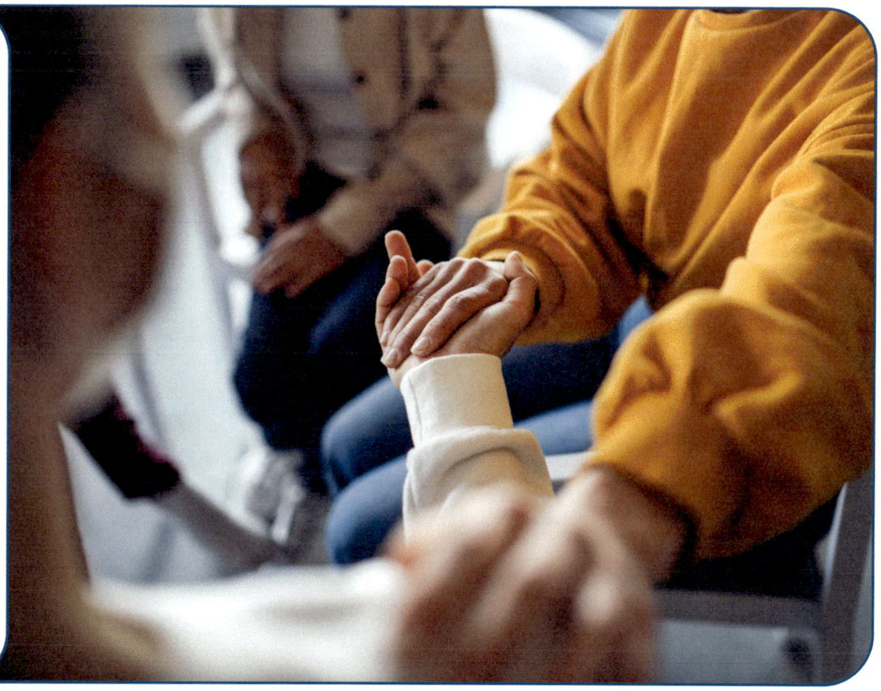

- RT
- Chemoradiation, **see Guide 6.**
- Clinical trial

Locally advanced

In locally advanced cancer, the tumor may be any size and cancer may be in 1 or more lymph nodes. The tumor might have grown into the larynx (voice box) or other nearby structures.

Treatment options for locally advanced cancer include:

- Chemoradiation (preferred in some cases), **see Guide 6.**
- Surgery to remove the tumor and lymph nodes. RT or chemoradiation, might follow surgery.
- Clinical trial

How throat cancer can spread

Cancer can spread to lymph nodes and other parts of the neck such as the base of the skull, epiglottis, larynx, pharynx, bones and muscles behind the nasal cavity, jaw, and roof of the mouth.

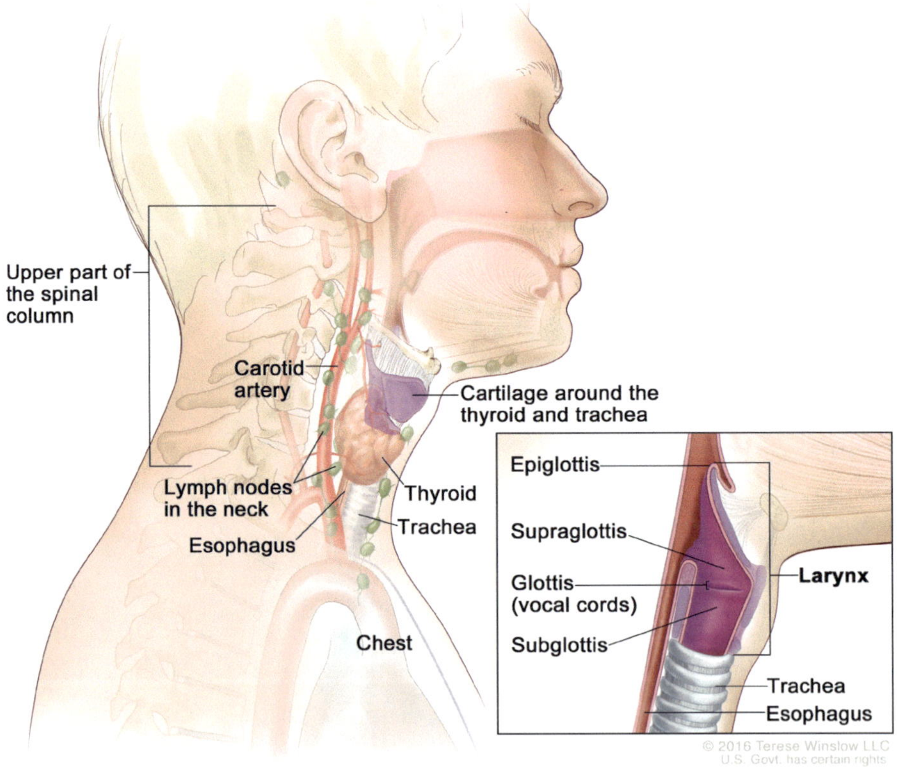

Follow-up care

After treatment, you will be monitored for side effects and the return of cancer called recurrence. General follow-up care includes doctor visits, blood and imaging tests, and supportive care as needed. It is important to contact your doctor right away if you notice any changes in your head or neck. For general follow-up care, **see Guide 7.**

Key points

- A p16-positive (p16+) throat cancer is caused by the HPV16 virus.
- In early-stage cancer, the tumor is 4 cm or less and cancer may be in 1 lymph node.
- In locally advanced cancer, the tumor may be any size and cancer may be in 1 or more lymph nodes. The tumor might have grown into the larynx (voice box) or other nearby structures.
- Treatment is based on the size and location of the tumor(s) and if there is cancer in the lymph nodes.
- After completing treatment, you will have follow-up care to monitor for sides effects and changes in your health. Contact your doctor right away if you notice any changes in your head or neck.

Warnings about supplements and drug interactions

You might be asked to stop taking or avoid certain herbal supplements when on a systemic therapy. Some supplements can affect the ability of a drug to do its job. This is called a drug interaction.

It is critical to speak with your care team about any supplements you may be taking. Some examples include:

- Turmeric
- Ginkgo biloba
- Green tea extract
- St. John's Wort
- Antioxidants

Certain medicines can also affect the ability of a drug to do its job. Antacids, heart or blood pressure medicine, and antidepressants are just some of the medicines that might interact with a systemic therapy or supportive care medicines given during systemic therapy. Therefore, it is very important to tell your care team about any medicines, vitamins, over-the-counter (OTC) drugs, herbals, or supplements you are taking.

Bring a list with you to every visit.

7 Advanced cancer

Advanced throat cancer is sometimes also called very advanced cancer. This is cancer that remains after treatment (persistent cancer) or cancer that has returned after a disease-free period (recurrence). It also includes cancer that cannot be removed with surgery (unresectable) or cancer that has spread to near (locoregional) or distant (metastatic) sites through the bloodstream. Together, you and your care team will choose a treatment plan that is best for you.

Tumor mutation or biomarker testing might be done before starting treatment for advanced or very advanced cancer. Ask how treatment will impact the quality of your life and if the goal is to cure or prevent the further spread of cancer.

Unresectable

An unresectable tumor cannot be removed with surgery. Sometimes, it is unsafe to remove the tumor with surgery because it is too close to vital organs. You may not want surgery. You may have other health conditions that prevent surgery. Treatment options are based on your performance status (PS) or your general level of fitness and ability to perform daily self-care tasks. Your preferences about treatment are always important.

Treatments like chemotherapy or radiation can cause an unresectable tumor to become resectable. This means that in some cases surgery might be possible in some unresectable cancers after chemoradiation, radiation therapy, or systemic therapy.

PS 0 or 1

A score of 0 means you are fully active. A score of 1 means you can do all self-care activities but are unable to do hard physical work.

For PS 0 or 1 (fully active), the options are:

- Chemoradiation
- Systemic therapy followed by radiation therapy or chemoradiation. The preferred systemic therapy is docetaxel with cisplatin and 5-FU. Paclitaxel with cisplatin and 5-FU is also an option.
- Radiation therapy

PS 2

A score of 2 means you can do most self-care tasks and spend most of waking time out of bed but are unable to do any work.

For PS 2, the options are:

- Chemoradiation (preferred)
- Radiation therapy

PS 3

A score of 3 means you need help with some self-care tasks and spend most of waking time in bed.

For PS 3, the options are:

- Palliative radiation therapy
- Systemic therapy, **see Guide 8**
- Best supportive care

Supportive care is health care given to prevent, reduce, and relieve suffering, and to improve quality of life. Best supportive care, supportive care, and palliative care are often used to mean the same thing.

Recurrent or persistent disease

Recurrent disease is cancer that has returned after a disease-free period. Persistent disease is cancer that remains after treatment. It might include cancer that has grown or spread during treatment, or is resistant to the treatment.

Recurrent or persistent disease treatment options are based on:

- If you had radiation therapy before, and
- If the tumor can be removed with surgery (resectable) or cannot be removed with surgery (unresectable).

Surgery is an option

A resectable tumor can be removed with surgery. If surgery is done, it might be followed by radiation therapy (RT), chemoradiation, or a clinical trial. A clinical trial is preferred in some cases. Surgery is not the only option for a resectable tumor, particularly if the surgery is anticipated to affect swallowing or speaking. In these cases, other options include chemoradiation or systemic therapy followed by RT or chemoradiation.

Surgery is not an option

An unresectable tumor cannot be removed with surgery because it is too close to vital organs. Sometimes, an unresectable tumor can become resectable after treatment. Treatment options include those on the previous page in the "Unresectable" section.

Guide 8
Systemic therapy options: Recurrent, unresectable, or metastatic disease

Preferred	First-line: • Pembrolizumab with platinum-based chemotherapy (cisplatin or carboplatin), and 5-FU • Pembrolizumab (for tumors that express PD-L1 with combined positive score of 1 or more)	Next-line (if not used before): • Nivolumab (if disease progresses on or after platinum-based chemotherapy) • Pembrolizumab (if disease progresses on or after platinum-based chemotherapy)
Other recommended	Combined drugs: • Cetuximab with platinum-based chemotherapy and 5-FU • Cisplatin with cetuximab • Platinum-based chemotherapy with docetaxel or paclitaxel • Cisplatin with 5-FU • Platinum-based chemotherapy with docetaxel and cetuximab • Platinum-based chemotherapy with paclitaxel and cetuximab • Pembrolizumab with platinum-based chemotherapy and docetaxel • Pembrolizumab with platinum-based chemotherapy and paclitaxel	Single drugs: • Cisplatin • Carboplatin • Paclitaxel • Docetaxel • 5-FU • Methotrexate • Cetuximab • Capecitabine • Afatinib (next-line only, if disease progresses on or after platinum-based chemotherapy)
Used in some cases	• Cetuximab with nivolumab • Cetuximab with pembrolizumab • Paclitaxel with cetuximab • Docetaxel with cetuximab • Pembrolizumab (for MSI-H, dMMR, or TMB-H tumors) • Cisplatin with pemetrexed (for PS 0 or PS 1) • Gemcitabine with paclitaxel • Nivolumab with ipilimumab (for tumors with combined positive score of 20 or more and first-line only)	

Note: A platinum-based chemotherapy is cisplatin or carboplatin

Metastatic disease

Metastatic disease is cancer that has spread through the bloodstream to distant areas of the body. A clinical trial is preferred for metastatic disease. Depending on your overall health, your ability to perform activities of daily living (ADLs), your preferences about treatment, and the location and number of metastases, treatment options also include systemic therapy, surgery, radiation therapy, or chemoradiation. Palliative surgery and palliative radiation therapy along with other types of supportive care might be given to relieve pain, discomfort, swallowing difficulties, and side effects caused by cancer. For systemic therapy options, **see Guide 8.**

Key points

- Advanced throat cancer or very advanced cancer is cancer that remains after treatment (persistent cancer) or cancer that has returned after a cancer-free period (recurrence). It also includes cancer that cannot be removed with surgery (unresectable) or cancer that has spread to near (locoregional) or distant (metastatic) sites through the bloodstream.
- Treatment is based on the size and location of the tumor(s), if there is cancer in the lymph nodes, and what treatment you had before. Your overall health and preferences about treatment are also important.
- A resectable tumor can be removed with surgery. An unresectable tumor cannot be removed with surgery because it is too close to vital organs. Sometimes an unresectable tumor can become resectable after treatment with chemoradiation, radiation therapy, or systemic therapy.
- Metastatic disease is cancer that has spread through the bloodstream to distant areas of the body. A clinical trial is preferred for metastatic disease.

8
Making treatment decisions

It's important to be comfortable with the cancer treatment you choose. This choice starts with having an open and honest conversation with your care team.

It's your choice

In shared decision-making, you and your care team share information, discuss the options, and agree on a treatment plan. It starts with an open and honest conversation between you and your care team. Treatment decisions are very personal. What is important to you may not be important to someone else.

Some things that may play a role in your decision-making:

- What you want and how that might differ from what others want
- Your religious and spiritual beliefs
- Your feelings about certain treatments
- Your feelings about pain or side effects
- Cost of treatment, travel to treatment centers, and time away from school or work
- Quality of life and length of life
- How active you are and the activities that are important to you

Think about what you want from treatment. Discuss openly the risks and benefits of specific treatments and procedures. Weigh options and share concerns with your care team. If you take the time to build a relationship with your care team, it will help you feel supported when considering options and making treatment decisions.

Second opinion

It is normal to want to start treatment as soon as possible. While cancer can't be ignored, there is time to have another doctor review your test results and suggest a treatment plan. This is called getting a second opinion, and it's a normal part of cancer care. Even doctors get second opinions!

Things you can do to prepare:

- Check with your insurance company about its rules on second opinions. There may be out-of-pocket costs to see doctors who are not part of your insurance plan.
- Make plans to have copies of all your records sent to the doctor you will see for your second opinion.

Support groups

Many people diagnosed with cancer find support groups to be helpful. Support groups often include people at different stages of treatment. Some people may be newly diagnosed, while others may be finished with treatment. If your hospital or community doesn't have support groups for people with cancer, check out the websites listed in this book.

Questions to ask

Possible questions to ask your care team are listed on the following pages. Feel free to use these questions or come up with your own. Be clear about your goals for treatment and find out what to expect from treatment.

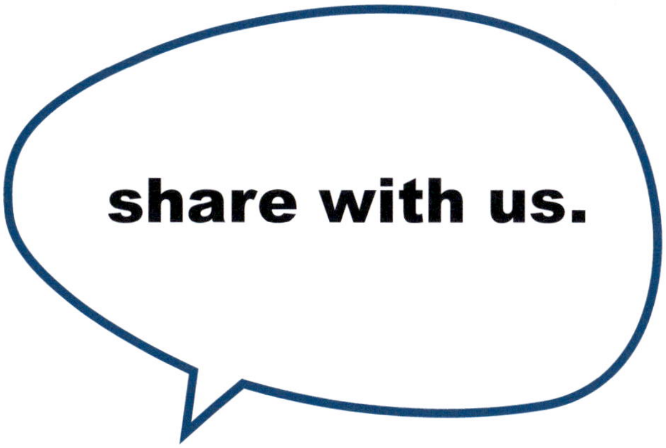

Take our survey, and help make the NCCN Guidelines for Patients better for everyone!

NCCN.org/patients/comments

Questions about testing and diagnosis

1. What tests will I have? How often will they be repeated?
2. Will my insurance pay for this test?
3. How soon will I know the results and who will explain them to me?
4. What will you do to make me comfortable during testing?
5. How will my biopsy be performed? What else might be done at this time?
6. Is my cancer resectable or unresectable? What does this mean?
7. Is the cancer early stage, locally advanced, advanced, or metastatic?
8. Is cancer in any other areas like my lymph nodes or lungs?
9. What does the cancer stage mean in terms of length of survival and quality of life?

Questions about your care team's experience

1. What is your experience treating this cancer? What else do you treat?
2. What is the experience of those on your team?
3. How many people like me (of the same age, gender, race) have you treated?
4. Will you be consulting with experts to discuss my care? Whom will you consult?
5. How many procedures like the one you're suggesting have you done?
6. Is this treatment a major part of your practice?
7. How many of your patients have had complications? What were the complications?
8. How many of these surgeries have you done?
9. Who will manage my day-to-day care?

Questions about options

1. What will happen if I do nothing?
2. How do my age, overall health, and other factors affect the options?
3. Which option is proven to work best for my cancer, age, overall health, and other factors?
4. What are the possible complications and side effects? Are any life-threatening?
5. What can be done to prevent or relieve the side effects of treatment?
6. Am I a candidate for a clinical trial? Can I join a clinical trial at any time?
7. What decisions must be made today?
8. Is there a social worker or someone who can help me decide about treatment?
9. Is there a hospital or treatment center you can recommend for treatment?
10. Can I go to one hospital for surgery and a different center for radiation therapy?

Questions about treatment

1. Which treatment(s) do you recommend and why?
2. Does the order of treatment matter?
3. When will I start treatment?
4. How long will treatment likely take?
5. What should I expect from treatment?
6. What will you do to make me comfortable during treatment?
7. How will treatment affect my ability to taste, smell, chew, breathe, talk, or swallow?
8. Can I work during treatment? When can I go back to work?
9. What are the chances my cancer will return after treatment?
10. I would like a second opinion. Is there someone you can recommend?

Questions about surgery

1. What will be removed during surgery?
2. How will surgery affect my ability to taste, smell, chew, breathe, talk, or swallow?
3. Does my cancer involve any veins, arteries, or nerves and how might this affect surgery?
4. Will I have or need more than one surgery?
5. Will I have reconstruction surgery after surgery to remove the tumor?
6. Will I have a scar and where will it be located?
7. How long will recovery take and what should I expect?
8. How much pain will I be in? What will be done to manage my pain?
9. What treatment will I have before, during, or after surgery?
10. How can I prepare for surgery and what to expect after surgery?

Questions about radiation therapy

1. What type of radiation therapy (RT) will I have?
2. What will you target?
3. What is the goal of this RT?
4. How many treatment sessions will I require? Can you do a shorter course of RT?
5. Do you offer this type of RT here? If not, should I be referred to someone who does?
6. What side effects can I expect from RT?
7. How will RT affect my ability to taste, smell, chew, breathe, talk, or swallow?
8. Should I eat or drink before RT?
9. Will I be given medicine to help me relax during RT?
10. What should I wear?

Questions about side effects

1. What are the side effects of this treatment?
2. How are these side effects treated?
3. How long will these side effects last?
4. What side effects should I watch for that could be life-threatening?
5. When should I call my care team?
6. What should I do on weekends and other non-office hours?
7. What emergency department or ER should I go to?
8. Will my treatment team be able to communicate with the ER team?
9. What medicines can I take to prevent or relieve side effects?
10. What can I do to help with pain and other side effects?

Questions about clinical trials

1. What clinical trials are available for my type and stage of cancer?
2. What are the treatments used in the clinical trial?
3. What does the treatment do?
4. Has the treatment been used before? Has it been used for other types of cancer?
5. What are the risks and benefits of this treatment?
6. What side effects should I expect? How will the side effects be controlled?
7. How long will I be in the clinical trial?
8. Will I be able to get other treatments if this doesn't work?
9. How will you know the treatment is working?
10. Will the clinical trial cost me anything? If so, how much?

Questions about resources and support

1. Who can I talk to about help with housing, food, and other basic needs?
2. What help is available for transportation, childcare, and home care?
3. How much will I have to pay for treatment?
4. What help is available to pay for medicines and treatment?
5. What other services are available to me and my caregivers?
6. How can I connect with others and build a support system?
7. How can I find in-person or online support?
8. Who can help me with my concerns about missing work or school?
9. Who can I talk to if I don't feel safe at home, at work, or in my neighborhood?
10. How can I get help to stop smoking or vaping?

Resources

Cancer Hope Network
Cancerhopenetwork.org

Head and Neck Cancer Alliance
Headandneck.org

HPV Cancers Alliance
hpvca.org

MedlinePlus
medlineplus.gov/cancers

MSI Insiders
msiinsiders.org

National Cancer Institute (NCI)
cancer.gov/types/head-and-neck

Oral Cancer Foundation
Oralcancerfoundation.org

Support for People with Oral and Head and Neck Cancers
Spohnc.org

THANC Foundation
Thancfoundation.org

Triage Cancer
triagecancer.org

Finding a clinical trial

In the United States

NCCN Cancer Centers
NCCN.org/cancercenters

The National Cancer Institute (NCI)
cancer.gov/about-cancer/treatment/clinical-trials/search

Worldwide

The U.S. National Library of Medicine (NLM)
clinicaltrials.gov

Need help finding a clinical trial?

NCI's Cancer Information Service (CIS)
1.800.4.CANCER (1.800.422.6237)
cancer.gov/contact

Words to know

biopsy
A procedure that removes fluid or tissue samples to be tested for a disease.

cancer burden
The amount or extent of cancer in the body.

cancer stage
A rating of the growth and spread of cancer.

carcinoma
Cancer that starts in cells that form the lining of organs and structures in the body.

chemotherapy
Drugs that kill cancer cells by damaging or disrupting the making of the genetic code.

clinical stage (c)
Rating the extent of a tumor based on tests before treatment.

clinical trial
Research on a test or treatment to assess its safety or how well it works.

computed tomography (CT)
A test that combines many x-rays to make pictures of the inside of the body.

contrast
A substance put into your body to make clearer pictures during imaging tests.

cricoid
The ring-shaped cartilage of the larynx.

cytology
The study of cells using a microscope.

distant recurrence
Cancer that has come back after treatment and is found in a part of the body far from the first (primary) tumor.

deoxyribonucleic acid (DNA)
A chain of chemicals in cells that contains coded instructions for making and controlling cells.

Eastern Cooperative Oncology Group (ECOG) Performance Scale
A rating scale of one's ability to do daily activities.

endoscope
A thin, long tube fitted with tools that is guided down the mouth.

epiglottis
A flap of tissue that closes when you eat or drink that prevents food and liquid from entering the windpipe (trachea).

first-line treatment
The first drug or set of drugs given to treat cancer.

gene
Coded instructions in cells for making new cells and controlling how cells behave.

histology
The structure of cells, tissue, and organs as viewed under a microscope.

imaging
A test that makes pictures (images) of the insides of the body.

immune system
The body's natural defense against infection and disease.

immunotherapy
A treatment with drugs that help the body find and destroy cancer cells.

interventional radiologist
A doctor who is an expert in imaging tests and using image-guided tools to perform minimally invasive techniques to diagnose or treat disease.

intravenous (IV)
A method of giving drugs by a needle or tube inserted into a vein.

Karnofsky Performance Status (KPS)
A rating scale of one's ability to do daily activities.

laryngoscope
A thin, long tube fitted with tools that is guided down the mouth to view the larynx (voice box).

local recurrence
Cancer that has come back after treatment in or near the same place as the first (primary) tumor.

lung function tests
Used to measure how well the lungs work. It measures how much air the lungs can hold and how quickly air is moved into and out of the lungs. It also measures how much oxygen is used and how much carbon dioxide is given off during breathing. Also called PFT and pulmonary function test.

lymph
A clear fluid containing white blood cells.

lymph node
A small group of disease-fighting cells located throughout the body.

lymph node dissection
A type of surgery that removes some disease-fighting structures called lymph nodes.

lymph vessels
Tubes that carry lymph—a clear fluid containing white blood cells that fight disease and infection—throughout the body and connect lymph nodes to one another.

magnetic resonance imaging (MRI)
A test that uses radio waves and powerful magnets to make pictures of the insides of the body.

medical oncologist
A doctor who's an expert in cancer drugs.

metastasis
The spread of cancer cells from the first tumor to another body part.

microsatellite instability (MSI)
Errors made in small, repeated DNA parts during the copy process because of an abnormal repair system.

microsatellite instability-high (MSI-H)
Mutations in 30% or more microsatellites.

mutation
An abnormal change.

nasopharynx
The part of the throat that is behind the nose.

neck dissection
An operation that removes lymph nodes and other tissue in the neck area.

oral cavity
Refers to the mouth. It includes the lips, the lining inside the cheeks and lips, the front two thirds of the tongue, the upper and lower gums, the floor of the mouth under the tongue, the bony roof of the mouth, and the small area behind the wisdom teeth.

oropharynx
The middle part of the throat.

palliative care
Treatment for symptoms of a disease. Also sometimes called supportive care.

palliative radiation
Radiation therapy used to relieve symptoms caused by the cancer.

palliative surgery
Surgery used to relieve symptoms caused by the cancer.

Panorex x-ray
A picture of the inside of the entire mouth, including the jaw.

pathologic stage (p)
A rating of the extent of cancer based on microscopic review after treatment.

pathologist
A doctor who's an expert in examining tissue and cells to find disease.

positron emission tomography (PET)
A test that uses radioactive material to see the shape and function of body parts.

primary treatment
The main treatment used to rid the body of cancer.

primary tumor
The first mass of cancer cells in the body.

prognosis
The likely course and outcome of a disease based on tests.

programmed death-ligand 1 (PD-L1)
An immune system protein found on some cancer cells.

radiation oncologist
A doctor who's an expert in radiation treatment.

radiation therapy (RT)
A treatment that uses high-energy rays.

radiologist
A doctor who is an expert in imaging tests.

radiotracer
A substance that releases small amounts of energy (radiation) that is put into the body to make pictures clearer.

recurrence
The return of cancer after a cancer-free period.

relapse
The return of cancer after treatment. Also called a recurrence.

resectable
Cancer that can be removed with surgery.

side effect
An unhealthy or unpleasant physical or emotional response to treatment

resection
Surgery to remove a tumor.

side effect
An unhealthy or unpleasant physical or emotional response to treatment.

staging
The process of rating and describing the extent of cancer in the body.

standard of care
The best-known way to treat a particular disease based on past clinical trials. There may be more than one treatment regimen that is considered standard of care.

stereotactic body radiation therapy (SBRT)
Radiation therapy given in higher doses to smaller areas over 1 to 5 sessions of treatment.

subtype
A smaller group within a type of cancer that is based on certain cell features as seen under a microscope.

supportive care
Health care that includes symptom relief but not cancer treatment. Also called palliative care and best supportive care.

surgical margin
The normal-looking tissue around the edge of a tumor removed during surgery.

surgical oncologist
A surgeon who's an expert in performing surgical procedures in those with cancer.

surveillance
Monitors for the return of cancer.

targeted therapy
Treatment with drugs that target a specific or unique feature of cancer cells.

throat
A hollow, muscular tube inside the neck that starts behind the nose and ends at the top of the trachea (windpipe) and esophagus (the tube that goes to the stomach).

treatment plan
A written course of action through cancer treatment and beyond.

tumor
An abnormal mass of cells.

ultrasound (US)
A test that uses sound waves to take pictures of the insides of the body.

unresectable
Cancer that can't be completely removed by surgery.

NCCN Contributors

This patient guide is based on the NCCN Clinical Practice Guidelines in Oncology (NCCN Guidelines®) for Head and Neck Cancers Version 1.2024. It was adapted, reviewed, and published with help from the following people:

Dorothy A. Shead, MS
Senior Director
Patient Information Operations

Tanya Fischer, MEd, MSLIS
Senior Medical Writer

Laura Phillips
Graphic Artist

The NCCN Clinical Practice Guidelines in Oncology (NCCN Guidelines®) for Head and Neck Cancers Version 1.2024 were developed by the following NCCN Panel Members:

David G. Pfister, MD
Memorial Sloan Kettering Cancer Center

*Sharon Spencer, MD
O'Neal Comprehensive Cancer Center at UAB

Douglas Adkins, MD
Siteman Cancer Center at Barnes-Jewish Hospital and Washington University School of Medicine

Andrew C. Birkeland, MD
UC Davis Comprehensive Cancer Center

David M. Brizel, MD
Duke Cancer Institute

Paul M. Busse, MD, PhD
Massachusetts General Hospital Cancer Center

Jimmy J. Caudell, MD, PhD
Moffitt Cancer Center

*Anthony J. Cmelak, MD
Vanderbilt-Ingram Cancer Center

A. Dimitrios Colevas, MD
Stanford Cancer Institute

Greg Durm, MD, MS
Indiana University Melvin and Bren Simon Comprehensive Cancer Center

*Carole Fakhry, MD, MPH
The Sidney Kimmel Comprehensive Cancer Center at Johns Hopkins

Thomas Galloway, MD
Fox Chase Cancer Center

Jessica L. Geiger, MD
Case Comprehensive Cancer Center/ University Hospitals Seidman Cancer Center and Cleveland Clinic Taussig Cancer Institute

Maura L. Gillison, MD, PhD
The University of Texas MD Anderson Cancer Center

Robert I. Haddad, MD
Dana-Farber/Brigham and Women'sCancer Center

Wesley L. Hicks, Jr., MD
Roswell Park Cancer Institute

Ying J. Hitchcock, MD
Huntsman Cancer Institute at the University of Utah

Antonio Jimeno, MD, PhD
University of Colorado Cancer Center

Debra Leizman, MD
Case Comprehensive Cancer Center/ University Hospitals Seidman Cancer Center and Cleveland Clinic Taussig Cancer Institute

Ellie Maghami, MD
City of Hope National Medical Center

Loren K. Mell, MD
UC San Diego Moores Cancer Center

Bharat B. Mittal, MD
Robert H. Lurie Comprehensive Cancer Center of Northwestern University

Harlan A. Pinto, MD
Stanford Cancer Institute

James W. Rocco, MD, PhD
The Ohio State University Comprehensive Cancer Center - James Cancer Hospital and Solove Research Institute

Cristina P. Rodriguez, MD
Fred Hutchinson Cancer Center

Panayiotis S. Savvides, MD, PhD
Mayo Clinic Comprehensive Cancer Center

David Schwartz, MD
The University of Tennessee Health Science Center

Jatin P. Shah, MD, PhD
Memorial Sloan Kettering Cancer Center

David Sher, MD, MPH
UT Southwestern Simmons Comprehensive Cancer Center

*Maie St. John, MD, PhD
UCLA Jonsson Comprehensive Cancer Center

He Wang, MD, PhD
Yale Cancer Center Smilow Cancer Hospital

Gregory Weinstein, MD
Abramson Cancer Center at the University of Pennsylvania

*Francis Worden, MD
University of Michigan Rogel Cancer Center

Justine Yang Bruce, MD
University of Wisconsin Carbone Cancer Center

Sue S. Yom, MD, PhD
UCSF Helen Diller Family Comprehensive Cancer Center

Weining Zhen, MD
Fred & Pamela Buffett Cancer Center

NCCN

Susan Darlow, PhD
Manager Guidelines Information Standardization

Nicole McMillian, MS
Senior Guidelines Coordinator

Sarah Montgomery, BA
Guidelines Layout Specialist

* Reviewed this patient guide. For disclosures, visit NCCN.org/disclosures.

NCCN Cancer Centers

Abramson Cancer Center
at the University of Pennsylvania
Philadelphia, Pennsylvania
800.789.7366 • pennmedicine.org/cancer

Case Comprehensive Cancer Center/
University Hospitals Seidman Cancer Center and
Cleveland Clinic Taussig Cancer Institute
Cleveland, Ohio
UH Seidman Cancer Center
800.641.2422 • uhhospitals.org/services/cancer-services
CC Taussig Cancer Institute
866.223.8100 • my.clevelandclinic.org/departments/cancer
Case CCC
216.844.8797 • case.edu/cancer

City of Hope National Medical Center
Duarte, California
800.826.4673 • cityofhope.org

Dana-Farber/Brigham and Women's Cancer Center |
Mass General Cancer Center
Boston, Massachusetts
617.732.5500 • youhaveus.org
617.726.5130 • massgeneral.org/cancer-center

Duke Cancer Institute
Durham, North Carolina
888.275.3853 • dukecancerinstitute.org

Fox Chase Cancer Center
Philadelphia, Pennsylvania
888.369.2427 • foxchase.org

Fred & Pamela Buffett Cancer Center
Omaha, Nebraska
402.559.5600 • unmc.edu/cancercenter

Fred Hutchinson Cancer Center
Seattle, Washington
206.667.5000 • fredhutch.org

Huntsman Cancer Institute at the University of Utah
Salt Lake City, Utah
800.824.2073 • healthcare.utah.edu/huntsmancancerinstitute

Indiana University Melvin and Bren Simon
Comprehensive Cancer Center
Indianapolis, Indiana
888.600.4822 • www.cancer.iu.edu

Mayo Clinic Comprehensive Cancer Center
Phoenix/Scottsdale, Arizona
Jacksonville, Florida
Rochester, Minnesota
480.301.8000 • Arizona
904.953.0853 • Florida
507.538.3270 • Minnesota
mayoclinic.org/cancercenter

Memorial Sloan Kettering Cancer Center
New York, New York
800.525.2225 • mskcc.org

Moffitt Cancer Center
Tampa, Florida
888.663.3488 • moffitt.org

O'Neal Comprehensive Cancer Center at UAB
Birmingham, Alabama
800.822.0933 • uab.edu/onealcancercenter

Robert H. Lurie Comprehensive Cancer Center
of Northwestern University
Chicago, Illinois
866.587.4322 • cancer.northwestern.edu

Roswell Park Comprehensive Cancer Center
Buffalo, New York
877.275.7724 • roswellpark.org

Siteman Cancer Center at Barnes-Jewish Hospital
and Washington University School of Medicine
St. Louis, Missouri
800.600.3606 • siteman.wustl.edu

St. Jude Children's Research Hospital/
The University of Tennessee Health Science Center
Memphis, Tennessee
866.278.5833 • stjude.org
901.448.5500 • uthsc.edu

Stanford Cancer Institute
Stanford, California
877.668.7535 • cancer.stanford.edu

The Ohio State University Comprehensive Cancer Center -
James Cancer Hospital and Solove Research Institute
Columbus, Ohio
800.293.5066 • cancer.osu.edu

The Sidney Kimmel Comprehensive
Cancer Center at Johns Hopkins
Baltimore, Maryland
410.955.8964
www.hopkinskimmelcancercenter.org

The UChicago Medicine Comprehensive Cancer Center
Chicago, Illinois
773.702.1000 • uchicagomedicine.org/cancer

The University of Texas MD Anderson Cancer Center
Houston, Texas
844.269.5922 • mdanderson.org

UC Davis Comprehensive Cancer Center
Sacramento, California
916.734.5959 • 800.770.9261
health.ucdavis.edu/cancer

UC San Diego Moores Cancer Center
La Jolla, California
858.822.6100 • cancer.ucsd.edu

UCLA Jonsson Comprehensive Cancer Center
Los Angeles, California
310.825.5268 • cancer.ucla.edu

UCSF Helen Diller Family
Comprehensive Cancer Center
San Francisco, California
800.689.8273 • cancer.ucsf.edu

University of Colorado Cancer Center
Aurora, Colorado
720.848.0300 • coloradocancercenter.org

University of Michigan Rogel Cancer Center
Ann Arbor, Michigan
800.865.1125 • rogelcancercenter.org

University of Wisconsin Carbone Cancer Center
Madison, Wisconsin
608.265.1700 • uwhealth.org/cancer

UT Southwestern Simmons
Comprehensive Cancer Center
Dallas, Texas
214.648.3111 • utsouthwestern.edu/simmons

Vanderbilt-Ingram Cancer Center
Nashville, Tennessee
877.936.8422 • vicc.org

Yale Cancer Center/Smilow Cancer Hospital
New Haven, Connecticut
855.4.SMILOW • yalecancercenter.org

Index

Made in United States
Troutdale, OR
08/06/2025

33427787R00052